# *What Others Are Saying about This Book...*

A powerful and shocking psychological drama reminiscent of the Academy Award-winning *A Beautiful Mind*. This true story will have you on the edge of your seat from beginning to end. Spellbinding! **—Josh Miller, Producer**

It is with great pleasure that I offer the foreword for a book that describes Christine's long and successful journey. It has been a joy to know and work with her. I hope that her book provides encouragement and strength to others in similar circumstances. Recovery is possible. **—Dr. Doug Jurgens, therapist**

Anyone who has ever questioned herself will find common ground in this stunning probe into the often secret landscape of the mind. There have been other books done on the topic of multiple personalities, but what makes this one special is that few therapists focus on integration as the best way to treat the patient (because of the rigor, time, and training involved). As one of Christine's therapists, the focus was on the integration of her alters—and we achieved it. **— Lynette Bushman, therapist**

Hers is an unimaginable journey, even to those of us who have suffered childhood trauma; but what a triumph for Christine Ducommun to emerge and share this extraordinary story! **—Jane Congdon, author of *It Started with Dracula: The Count, My Mother, and Me***

This chilling, but tender, book has been ten years in the making. When Christine first contacted me a decade ago asking if I would help her bring her book to light, working on it revealed she still had

D1545853

much work to do in her treatment and care. Now on the other side of this intense regimen, Christine shines a bright light not only on her spectacular journey into and out of Disassociative Identity Disorder, but on the fragility of the human mind and the immense durability of the human spirit. We look forward to this book, and the upcoming film it has inspired. **—Bettie Youngs, Publisher**

An incredible story; a courageous journey; an unforgettable memoir. **—Ron Russell, author of *DON CARINA***

This riveting personal memoir will appeal to those wishing to better understand the power of the human psyche. Part mystery and part survival story, this unforgettable book is ultimately a story of the strength of the mind and spirit from which we can all find encouragement to walk through the fire of our own lives. **—Christine Belleris, editor, *Living With Multiple Personalities***

A special book, a beautiful book. **—Aura Imbarus, author of *Out of the Transylvania Night***

Christine's book is proof positive that while we humans are tender and fragile beings, when we venture into the land of courage, we are powerfully resilient and can endure even the most arduous of journeys. Congratulations Christine, on showing us the warrior's spirit that resides within our souls. **—William Chasey, author of *Truth Never Dies***

Christine's book is an incredible story that offers hope in times of darkness, and encouragement in that it bears out that peace comes through the healing journey. **—Charmaine Hammond, author of *On Toby's Terms***

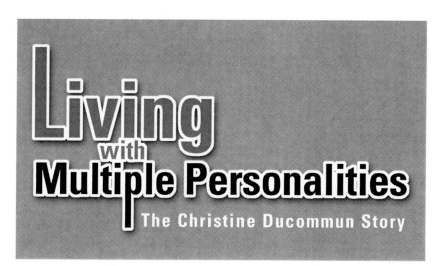

# Living
## with
# Multiple Personalities
### The Christine Ducommun Story

Christine Ducommun

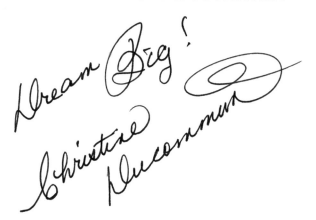

Dream Big!
Christine Ducommun

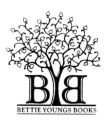

BETTIE YOUNGS BOOKS

Disclaimer: This is a true story, and the characters and events are real. However, in some cases, the names, descriptions, and locations have been changed, and some events have been altered, combined, or condensed for storytelling purposes, but the overall chronology is an accurate depiction of the author's experience.

Cover design by Tatomir Pitarui and Jane Hagaman
Text design by Jane Hagaman

Bettie Youngs Books are distributed worldwide. If you are unable to order this book from your local bookseller or online or Espresso, you may order directly from the publisher.

BETTIE YOUNGS BOOK PUBLISHERS
www.BettieYoungsBooks.com

ISBN: 978-0-9843081-5-6

Library of Congress Control Number: 2010915365
1. Ducommun, Christine. 2. Dissociative Identity Disorder (DID) 3. Mental health. 4. Family Relationships 5. Self-image 6. Sexual abuse 7. Inner Child

10 9 8 7 6 5 4 3 2 1

Printed on acid-free paper

# Contents

# Foreword

Agreeing to write the foreword for this book caused me to review both Christine's and my own journey with dissociative identity disorder (DID). My training did not focus on helping people with what was then called multiple personality disorder (MPD). Indeed, it was more common to debate whether the disorder existed at all than to discuss treatment methods. What I was taught and was able to find in my own review of the literature suggested that the therapist should determine which one of the personalities was the "core" or primary personality and direct most efforts to assisting this personality. It was thought that the other personalities were less important and "complete" than the core personality and, indeed, were termed "alters" in much of what I was taught and read. Somehow the alters would eventually agree to "die" or to stop taking executive control of the body. I could not see how they would agree to do so. There was a significant lack of research into the topic due largely to the disorder's rarity and to doubts amongst researchers and clinicians of its existence. Therefore, there was no evidence-based manner in which I could see to proceed. The prevailing theories about how to treat patients with DID did not strike me as sensible. I was not clear on how I should proceed to assist these people. This did not sit well with me.

I first became aware of Christine Ducommun when her therapist at the time contacted me for a consultation. She described an adult woman who was manifesting a child personality and wondered whether it would be potentially harmful to engage in play therapy with the patient in the child persona. While not certain in my response, it seemed sensible to me that if a child personality would be more comfortable receiving therapy in a play setting that it would likely not harm her. What my training did very well was encourage me to focus on the person in therapy and to provide the safest and most comfortable environment that I could in order to facilitate personal exploration. It was with this in mind that I recommended play therapy for the child personality.

Christine's therapist consulted with me regarding her care a few more times before she ultimately retired, leaving Christine without a treatment provider. It was also around that time that Christine was charged with criminal offenses that were committed by another of her personalities. It was in this context that I agreed to become her primary therapist.

Early visits were focused on the establishment of trust and the creation of a safe and comfortable treatment setting. It was difficult for Christine to trust anyone at that time, much less a large and imposing man in a position of authority. Rather than use prevailing theories on treating DID, I determined to treat each of her personalities as complete people unto themselves. That is, while I recognized that none of Christine's personalities could be considered complete, functional people as each had a specific set of skills and abilities while almost completely lacking others, each still needed to be valued as individuals. For me it was a matter of respect. In fact, I determined to call each of her personalities "selves", rather than "alters", and to treat each as if they were separate patients. This approach seemed sensible to me and was well-received by Christine.

Once I became familiar with most of the selves that made up Christine's dissociative system, the task became to increase cooperation amongst them. DID is associated with powerful amnestic barriers between many of the selves. Some individuals within the system feel unable to manage certain kinds of situations, for example, an angry confrontation. When faced with an angry confrontation, people with DID "switch" to a self who is more comfortable and able to manage such situations. In this way, individuals in the system are able to avoid situations that cause them to feel fear or discomfort. I encouraged Christine's selves to share experiences. That is, I encouraged selves to "look through the eyes" of the self who was in control at the time so that they would be exposed to a wider range of experiences and so that they would learn that they could tolerate and manage emotions and could share skills amongst themselves. In this way, selves could gain mastery and confidence.

Finally, it was important for misunderstandings and conflicts amongst the selves to be mediated. With strong amnestic barriers there is the potential for powerful mistrust. The actions of some selves are difficult for other selves to accept, for example aggressive, criminal or sexual behavior to a highly moral and virtuous self. This can contribute to selves opposing and demonizing other selves. In Christine's care it was important to help her selves to recognize that each self has an equal right to exist and an equal right to determine their own course in life. As the selves shared experiences by looking through each other's eyes, the need for amnestic barriers decreased and differences between the selves gradually diminished until we were left with a single individual, Christine.

It is with great pleasure that I offer this foreword to a book that describes Christine's long and successful journey. It has been a joy to know and work with her. I hope that her book provides encouragement and strength to others in similar circumstances. Recovery is possible.

*–Douglas Jurgens, Ph.D.*

# Acknowledgments

I want to give my deepest gratitude to the following people who made this book possible:

First and foremost, I would like to thank two wonderful therapists, Lynette and Doug, for their tenacity and insight into a mental disorder many chose to ignore.

To family and friends, old and new, who had what it took to believe that this could be done and to those who helped me financially. It has sometimes been a rough ride; thanks for hanging on, even when I tried to let go.

To my publisher's cast of brilliant talent: To two fantastic editors, Elisabeth Rinaldi and the incomparable Christine Belleris, for their kindness and wisdom in handling such an emotional subject, for their professionalism and their uncanny way of drawing just a little extra from me; to Jane Hagaman for the beautiful attention to detail on the interior and back cover design of this book; and to Tatomir Pitariu for an amazing cover. Thank you, all.

Last but not least, to Bettie Youngs, whom I first contacted over ten years ago. I had finished only twenty-three pages of this book manuscript and was overwhelmed. I didn't think I could do it. I finished reading one of the *Chicken Soup for the Soul* books in which Bettie was a beloved contributor. Her words offered such encouragement I decided to write her, with a hope and prayer she might answer. I didn't have to wait long and she did, saying this was a story that should be told, and she encouraged me to continue and to get a computer. I put the letter and the book manuscript away for several years. Finally, I did get it out and the timing was right; everything flowed naturally. When I finished—I had a computer now—I emailed Bettie asking her if she remembered me. She did remember my story—and me. The rest has been a fantastic learning experience as she has mentored me through every edit both as my publisher and my friend. Her energy, wisdom and compassion have been inspirational.

# Introduction

When I moved back to my childhood home with my husband and family, I envisioned a time of great promise. I was thirty-eight, happily married, with two young sons. Instead, this move was the catalyst for a turbulent twelve-year odyssey of discovering a horrific past, reaching the brink of madness, and—with much hard work and determination—returning to sanity and a whole life.

I was diagnosed with dissociative identity disorder (DID), a psychological condition that develops as a reaction to childhood trauma. Specifically, an individual's response to being severely traumatized as a young child is to wall off, in other words, to dissociate those memories. In my case, my mind had created—in addition to me—five distinct personalities, or alters, to help me cope with trauma in my early years.

What follows is my story and that of the five personalities who came to be called the Board of Directors, and how each fought to become the Chief Executive Officer of my mind. And, oh my, what characters they were! One strapped me with legal woes and criminal charges while another lead me to seek treatment for chemical dependency. One made a decision about the man I would marry, and another became the strongest front and friend any gal could hope for.

It is with much humility and a bit of trepidation that I share this very personal journey of growing up with the cast of characters who worked to protect me as a child—but who, in adulthood, struggling for control of my mind, spiraled my life into unimaginable chaos, leaving me to believe I would lose the battle for my sanity.

Writing was cathartic. In the beginning, I had no intention of ever sharing what I was writing with anyone but my therapist. Later, it was a way of keeping track of time and, much later, it became a way for the five personalities to communicate with each other and with my therapist. But slowly, the journaling began to serve a more valuable lesson: it allowed me to track my progress, and chart a plan for wellness. As the therapy process progressed and more and more healing was achieved, and I had a growing desire to tell others of this incredulous journey.

The more I wrote, the more I shared my story with others—women in particular. Rather than finding me "odd," many shared stories about their own sense of mental health, from "I can't tell the difference between intuition and the strong directives in my head" to disclosing their own childhood trauma that derailed them in adult life. Some told me of their own diagnosis of DID, and others said that while not diagnosed, they were sure they had multiple personalities operating within themselves. Perhaps my story will give you the courage to go check out any "voices" in your head.

Ultimately I wrote this book because I am grateful. Grateful for ever member of my Board, an elaborate system created to protect an innocent child. Even when my life went strangely amiss in my adult years these characters in my head—these alters—helped me not only survive my childhood, but cope with the years of work that lie ahead.

It is my desire that all who read this book find hope and encouragement in the pages.

—*Christine Ducommun*

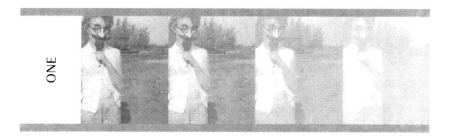

# ONE

## Back Where It All Began

I bolted up in my bed, terrified. Maybe it was a nightmare that woke me up so suddenly, but I had no recollection of it. I had kicked off the covers but was enveloped by a thick blanket of foreboding and dread. I surveyed the room, my eyes adjusting quickly because of the bright moonlight flowing through the huge east windows. It must be a full moon or close to it, I thought. Everything was so peaceful, so quiet, except for the hum of the bedside digital clock that glowed an eerie green and read 2:00 AM. My husband's breathing was slow and rhythmic and my two sons appeared to be sleeping as well. It couldn't have been a noise that had awakened me so suddenly or they would have heard it as well.

Ever so carefully I slid from the bed, not wanting to wake my husband. I trembled as I started down the thick-carpeted stairs. I clutched the soft pink terrycloth robe tightly to my body, hoping to stop the shaking. I was almost numb with terror, expecting someone or something to jump out from the shadows. Slowly, I made my way down the stairs, counting each one; every step deliberate, as if I wasn't quite sure the next stair was going to be there.

I finally made it to the middle of the living room, still clutching my robe tightly to my chest, still shaking. The bright, white moonlight washed over me. Ordinarily I would have appreciated its beauty but tonight the shimmering light gave everything an evil feeling. Here, in my own home, nothing felt safe. I wanted to hide, but I didn't know where—I didn't even know what it was I needed to hide from. I summoned all my strength to hold back the screams that welled up in my throat.

I felt like I was on the brink of a breakdown. How could this be happening to me? Life was so perfect but now I was terrified, desperately searching for some answers. "What is happening to me?" I pleaded silently.

This was not the first time this had happened to me. The episodes had started in the late autumn, about five months or so earlier, not long after my father had died. Each time, I would awaken in the middle of the night with this haunting, unsettling feeling—no nightmares, no noise, no apparent trigger that I could think of—just a dreadful feeling. I hadn't told anyone about this. Who would understand? I had never heard of this happening to anyone.

I wasn't haunted only at night. I'd also had terrible, unexplained mood swings during the day. They were precipitated by the feeling that someone was watching me, like I was in imminent danger. Most of the time I was content. I'd be happily painting, wall-papering and giving the house my feel and touch. Then it would suddenly roll in like a summer thunderstorm: I was instantly afraid and overwhelmed. I'd respond by getting cranky and short with my family. The guilt afterward was so consuming that I would hide in the bathroom, trying to cry it out of me, with a heavy towel over my face to muffle the anguish.

It had been six months since my husband, Rick, and I had moved our family into my childhood home where I had been raised. I was thirty-eight then and we had two young sons: Craig, who was five, and Cory, who was two. My husband had always wanted to live in the country, always dreamed of being a farmer. Leaving town for a rural life seemed like such a good idea at the time, and was a financial lifesaver to boot.

We were in the trucking business but had lost two major contracts. Backed into a corner, we were going to be forced to sell the business' assets. We had not told any of our family any of this. The family that was currently living on the home farm acreage and was also a member of the same church we went to was interested in trading the property to us for our semi-truck, truck shop and townhome. It seemed like an amazing coincidence: the subject had come up at coffee after a Bible study we attended together. We really hadn't decided for sure how we were going to handle the sale of the business and had no inclination of ever living there so this arrangement just seemed too perfect to pass up. Rick already had a job lined up with a local farmer so we went ahead with the deal. We actually waited till the paperwork was signed and we knew when we were moving to tell my family.

Rick and I were both excited to have this news to tell and I thought for sure my parents would be equally excited. "Mom, Dad, we have some news." I said. My dad had been diagnosed with cancer and was in failing health. He was groggy and laying on one of the sofas in the living room. Mom came in the living room from the kitchen.

"What kind of news?" Mom asked.

Rick was silent. "I think you'll be happy for us" I replied. Dad had raised himself up on one arm and proceeded to sit up.

"We have bought our home place, the farm sight," I said.

It became very quiet; no one said anything for a few seconds. Dad leaned back. Mom sat down.

It was awkward. I began to babble to fill in the void. "We have lost two big contracts and are forced to sell, and they wanted to trade us for the truck and the house in town. It is a really good deal for us and the kids will love the farm. Dad, we can drive you out to see it. The yard is a mess and needs some clean up, but we can do that and there is a big red hip-roof barn there now. Rick is looking into raising some cattle." Out of breath, I stopped talking.

"It's a big move," Mom said. "I will make us a coffee." Then she went back in the kitchen.

"Would you like to drive out and see it?" I asked Dad again.

"I don't think so," he whispered. "Your mom has ruined every good memory I have of that place."

I wasn't really sure I had heard him correctly and Mom was coming back in the room so I left it. We all left it. Nothing was mentioned to Dad again and he was dead a couple months later.

I just shrugged off their strange reaction. To me, this turn of events seemed predestined; like this was where God wanted me to raise my children. With six acres of land, there was lots of room for the boys to play, build tree forts and have pets. I could even grow a nice garden. The acreage had a big hip-roof barn and even some corral space, so we talked about raising some livestock.

The house was the perfect family home. It was solid, well-built and spacious. White clapboard with black-trimmed windows, it was constructed in the early 1950s by a local carpenter who crafted it for his family. Sadly, the carpenter passed away shortly after he had finished it, so his wife and daughters sold it and moved to town. My parents purchased it in 1959, and had it moved onto our yard right after our little house that Dad had built had burned down. This home had two stories, with the kitchen and dining area on the main floor and a large living room. There were four rooms on the second floor: a large master bedroom, two smaller bedrooms and a tiny room that was the perfect craft room/office. It also had a half-finished full basement, the completed part of which made an excellent playroom for Craig and Cory.

I loved the house because it had large windows that made it bright and cheery. It was set in a very pretty yard with a natural growth boreal forest running along the entire north side right behind the house. When the season was right you could find an abundance of wild flowers here, tiger lilies, bluebells, and marsh marigolds along with wild raspberries and strawberries.

It didn't trouble me that I had almost no memory of my childhood here. Sometimes I did wonder if that was normal, if other people didn't remember growing up. I was too busy to ask these questions of myself. When I did think about it, it was like I had arrived on the planet at age eleven.

❦

After what seemed like an eternity, the terror had finally passed and so I made my way back up the stairs. Quietly I slipped between the sheets, snuggling into my sleeping husband, trying to draw some solace from his warm, relaxed body. The moonlight infused the farmhouse with strange shadows and shapes, but no bother; I soon fell into a peacefully deep, sweet sleep.

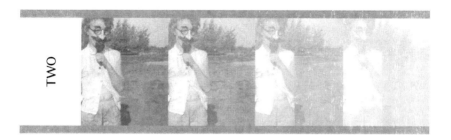

# TWO

## Rooted in the Soil

I grew up on a farm in central Saskatchewan on the edge of a huge natural forest. My paternal grandfather—originally from the French-speaking part of Switzerland—his wife, three children and four of his brothers, moved to this area of Canada in the early 1930s. The Great Depression and several years of drought on the prairie in southern Saskatchewan drove many farmers north to farm the heavily treed land. These pioneers cleared many acres by hand or were aided by horses. It was backbreaking work but they were rewarded with fertile, productive farmland.

My father was seven years old when they moved here. As soon as he was old enough to help, Dad began farming with his father. Since he was the only boy in the family, it was assumed he would take over the farm from my grandfather when the time came and that his sisters would get married and move out.

My mom also came from the same area on the prairie that Dad had and was working in a restaurant with Dad's sister when they met. Mom's father had abandoned his family during the Depression and reportedly had serious mental health issues. All of her family, which consisted of three brothers and five sisters, had left home at very young ages to fend for themselves.

Dad and Mom were married in 1949 when Mom was seventeen and Dad was twenty-three. They had four daughters: I was the oldest and born in 1952; Jan was born in 1956; Tess in 1962; and Laurie in 1966.

Our family farm was nearly self-supporting and we depended on the outside world for very little in the way of staples. We raised cattle, pigs and chickens. The pigs gave us meat. The chickens gave us meat and eggs. The cows gave us meat and milk.

In our huge garden we grew potatoes, peas, corn, tomatoes and cucumbers, which we'd also turn to pickles and relish. This was before the advent of large freezers so we'd preserve the harvested produce for consumption in the winter months by canning it. Shelves lined the basement, filled top to bottom with an assortment of canned vegetables and even canned chicken and beef.

On the crop land we grew wheat, oats, barley and hay, some for feeding the animals and some for sale to fill in the gaps.

Our farm was nearly ten miles from the closest town. Although it was very small, it provided all that we needed at the time. It had a grocery store, dry goods store, a pub, a café, doctor, even a theater that was built in the early sixties. It was a very close-knit community of farm folk from a kaleidoscope of nations: the Ukraine, Germany, Great Britain, France and Switzerland. Some had come to Canada through the United States. Saturday night was the time when all the families went into town together. The stores stayed open late. People would get groceries and visit with one another. The kids would go to a show and many of the men would gather in the pub, which was off-limits to women. It's hard to believe now, but until 1957 women were actually banned from entering a drinking establishment. This was in a rural area of Canada, newly developed, and slow to catch up with the times in some ways. There were times that Dad would get carried away and stay in the pub too long while Mom, and my younger sister Jan and I waited in the car. This was certainly not fun. All the stores were closed at 9 PM and the show was usually over around then, but the bar did not close until midnight. At best the ride home would be very quiet; at worst it was a shouting fest between Mom and Dad.

This was an extremely hard-working community and for the most part many played as hard as they worked. Apart from drinking at the pub there were several "home brewers" in the area, providing the harshest moonshine possible. People often had parties in their houses and dances were frequently held at the schoolhouses. Local artists provided the live music: piano, violin, guitar, and often accordion.

The adults weren't the only ones who worked hard on these small farms. Everyone had to pitch in. I grew up toiling alongside my sister and parents from the time I was very young, perhaps eight. I learned how to milk the cows and that is one of the first jobs I remember doing, along with feeding chickens. There were chores to be done in the morning before school and in the evening after getting home.

We rode the school bus, which picked us up around 8:15 every morning. I loved school. I loved learning. I loved new friends. It quickly became my favorite thing.

I was physically very strong because of all the farm work and I soon became very competitive, especially with the boys. I aimed to be better than them at anything they could do: track and field, softball, even arm wrestling. Getting good grades was also very important. Hard work and good grades seemed to get me praise, especially from my dad.

I really don't have many memories from early elementary school but I do recall that at about grade five boys began to appeal to me in a different way and I to them. Puberty came early for the women in our family and I was no exception. I acquired a curvy figure very young, not that I really cared at first because I was still focused on sports.

The first time I really felt like a girl was in grade seven. We were taught how to dance properly and had school dances. I really liked the feeling I got when I was in a boy's arms. By fourteen I was dating—which is when I had sex with a date for the first time. There was no discussion; I did what he wanted. Saying "no" hadn't even been a consideration. I quickly became very popular with the guys.

However, this led me to an unhappy realization: the same guys who wanted to date me and have sex with me were ignoring me everywhere else. Many, many times after a date would drop me off I would curl up in my bed and cry.

At sixteen I decided I needed a steady boyfriend; most all my friends had one. More than anything I wanted to get married. This was when I was introduced to Rick. He worked with a guy who was dating one of my friends and they set us up. He was five years older than I was, had a nice car, worked, had his own money and liked to party and have sex. It was 1968—a time of relaxed morality, Woodstock, and drugs, sex and rock 'n' roll—so this was not so out of line with what a lot of people were doing. His idea of pleasing me was buying the beer and getting me in the back seat. That worked for me because I didn't know anything else anyway. Besides, it was a woman's job to please the man and he *did* want to be with me. There was no doubt about that. We seemed perfect for each other. Quickly we became a steady couple and I found that, besides partying and having sex, we had many other similar interests, like fishing, hunting and snowmobiling. The next three years were full of that and we were inseparable.

I graduated from high school in 1970 and Rick and I were married in 1971, on my nineteenth birthday. It was the fulfillment of my wish and I thought that my prayers were answered. I was ecstatic; I truly believed I would now be happy.

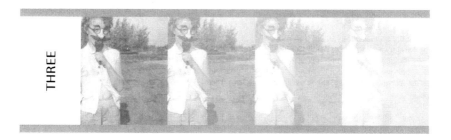

# THREE

# Sex, Rock 'n' Roll, and Rick

My early married years were spent in a haze. Most weekends we drank at house parties or bar-hopped from small town to small town. With no designated sober driver we put ourselves and everyone on the roads at great risk. The inebriation muffled the problems brewing in my marriage. Rick started to get very controlling. This was the way my parents' marriage operated so it was not alien to me: the man makes all the important decisions and the woman's role is to create an attractive home, have children and say "yes" to everything her husband demands of her, no matter how demeaning or ridiculous.

Soon Rick started spending more and more time drinking without me. Instead of coming home right after work, he'd head to the bar and stay for a couple of hours. This caused a lot of conflict between us and our arguments most often revolved around his right to keep his old friends.

Eight months after our wedding Rick lost his job. We decided to move to Alberta because there were more jobs available there at the time. Our luck was not much better there. Rick did find work but soon after had major health problems and couldn't work. He was beset with bleeding ulcers and had to have surgery on his stomach.

His doctors warned him to quit drinking or face even more serious consequences. This frightened him into stopping but only for about two months. I had started working but was not making a big salary and we could not make ends meet on one paycheck.

We decided that living in a bigger city might give us more opportunity to get better paying jobs, so we opted to move back to Saskatchewan; not to our home town but to Saskatoon, a larger center of about five hundred thousand people. We both soon had full-time jobs: Rick at a transmission shop and me at a department store. While this alleviated our financial problems it conversely propelled us into a vicious drinking cycle. I often drove to Rick's work because most days the men stayed after hours and drank. The manager at this transmission shop, which was almost entirely staffed by young men, would reward a good day's work by supplying a forty-ounce bottle of whiskey for his men. There were also several hard-core drinkers among the staff where I worked and, with a bar located in the same shopping mall as the store, it seemed natural to end the day there. Sometimes Rick would meet me and some of my co-workers for cocktails.

We both drank too much; nearly every day of the week and then more on weekends. I began to see this was getting out of control. We never missed work and I never had black-outs but waking up most days with a hangover got old after a while. There began to be a very obvious split between my drinking style and Rick's. I could stop before I got totally drunk but he didn't seem to be able to do that. I wasn't having a great time anymore and I began to look around at others, people I worked with; not all of them drank even on weekends much less during the week.

We wanted to buy a home and I knew at the rate we were spending money in this drinking lifestyle that wasn't going to happen, so I suggested we slow down. Surprisingly Rick agreed with me and for a month or so it did slow down. At this point I had given up alcohol altogether. But my optimism was short-lived. Soon Rick developed a new but familiar pattern of hanging out at bars after hours and drinking without me. He'd seldom come home sober.

I began trying to control that, sometimes by joining him and trying to talk him into leaving. If Rick said, "Why don't you stay and order something for yourself," I would remind him, "But remember, we're trying to save up for our house. Let's leave now before we spend too much." Sometimes that tactic worked, which gave me hope that I could fix this problem. More often, my pleas fell on deaf ears as Rick ignored me and ordered another round. I felt totally deflated and betrayed. *There has to be a way to make him stop drinking,* I thought, determined not to fail.

I orchestrated several moves to different parts of the city hoping that this would somehow precipitate a change and make the drinking stop but the vicious cycle continued for two years. Whenever I thought I had a handle on Rick's problem he would start again. Finally I decided we needed to become a family. I believed that having children would fill the void for Rick and he would give up alcohol. I thought that moving away from Saskatoon altogether, back to our little hometown, would do us some good. To my surprise, Rick agreed with all these things.

Right after our move, starting our family was the first order of business. We had been married for nearly four years at this point and, other than the three months at the beginning of our marriage, we had not used any birth control. We were pretty sure something was wrong so we sought professional help to diagnosis the problem. I was certain that we would quickly find an answer. We both endured a battery of undignified testing that revealed I couldn't conceive because of what appeared to be massive scarring and an undeveloped reproductive area. The doctors also determined Rick had an abnormally low sperm count. I felt inadequate, a failure, I blamed myself. Rick blamed himself. It was a blow to both of us, we were completely disheartened. The doctors didn't offer an explanation for either condition and we didn't ask. It was so painful and shameful that we never spoke about this to anyone else—or, for that matter, even to each other.

We decided to start adoption procedures. We waited for the miracle baby to arrive, a little child on whose tiny shoulders I rested a big task: getting Rick to grow up and settle down. I prayed that the added responsibilities of being a father would change him. God only knows the drinking had done nothing but escalate since our move back home, giving Rick renewed contact with his old buddies.

Two and a half years after our initial application, we were thrilled to learn that we would have a baby girl. The social worker told us that her biological parents were only teen-agers—in grade eleven—and had decided together that she would have a better life if she were put up for adoption.

I will never forget the feeling of anticipation and excitement I had on the day we traveled to pick her up. I assumed that Rick felt the same way.

"I wonder what she will look like," I said. "I am nervous; I hope I am a good mom. Are you nervous?"

Rick answered, "I sure am. And you *will* be a good mom, I just know you will." Most of the five-hour trip to Regina was quiet. We were both lost in our own thoughts of how our lives were going to change. I stared out the window dreaming of holding my little girl and starting our new life together.

When we finally arrived and I got to see her in person for the first time, she was just as I had pictured her. Only two-and-a-half months old, she was a healthy but delicate little girl, with wispy blonde hair, pale blue eyes and lovely soft pink skin. "Hello Roseanne," I cooed as I took her in my arms. "Welcome to your new family."

Looking at Rick I exclaimed, "She is perfect, we have a beautiful daughter!"

His eyes were misty and he looked like he might cry. In a very soft shaky voice he answered, "A daughter, we have a daughter."

After the long drive back, the thrill of having a child was mixed in with abject fear. I had no idea what I was doing and I was terrified. Luckily, my mother was a huge help. This was her first grandchild and so Roseanne was very special to her. My mother-in-law had given birth to fifteen children and had over twenty-five grandchildren by this time, so she was not interested in babysitting or much in the way of help.

I soon settled into the routine of being a mother, and I loved every minute of it. Looking at the baby took my breath away; she was so sweet and delicate. Even though I had not given birth to her she was mine and, for the first time in my life, I felt a love that was boundless. Roseanne gave me a sense of purpose. I wanted to be the best mom possible. I dreamed of what she would look like as she grew up and the things we would do together.

I joyfully cared for Roseanne but most days I did it alone. I had placed so much hope in this little sweetheart—not only as the key to my happiness, but a real reason for Rick to stop drinking. Sadly, I soon realized the latter was just a pipe dream. Rick seemed very pleased and proud of Roseanne but nothing, not even the responsibility of a new baby, was strong enough to lure him away from alcohol. Not long after we brought her home he quickly slipped back into his routine of hitting the bar after work. Seven years of marriage and it seemed like nothing would ever change him. I didn't want to acknowledge the emptiness of the dark house, where I would get anxious and upset. Instead I found peace in a smaller space: in my car, driving the country roads with my baby. It is one place I have always felt relaxed and Roseanne liked being in the car too. If she was fussy, it would always calm her down. I'd turn on the radio and we would drive for hours—especially all those many evenings Rick was in the bar. With Roseanne, I didn't feel alone anymore; I had a darling daughter to keep me company. For seven blissful months she was my world. Then it all came crashing down around me.

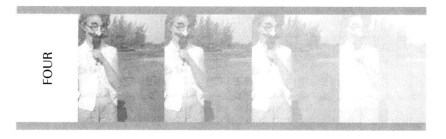

FOUR

# Another Angel in Heaven

It started out like any other day. Rick had gone to work a couple hours earlier. I fed Roseanne breakfast and gave her a morning bath. She was a week short of being ten months old and I marveled at how much she had changed since we first got her. She played in her walker for a while and then on the floor with her toys. I gave her a snack and put her down for a midmorning nap—a regular part of her routine.

The phone rang. "Hi Christine, is it okay if I come over for a visit?" It was Rick's mom.

"Sure," I answered, "I'd love to see you. Roseanne is napping but why don't you come over now anyway and we can chat over coffee." Rick's mother didn't drive so her husband dropped her off and I invited both of them in. While my mother-in-law was anxious to see the baby, Roseanne was still asleep when my father-in-law said he had to go. "Don't worry about leaving now," I said to Rick's mom, grateful for the adult conversation. "Why don't you stay and I can drive you home sometime before lunch?"

We talked for a long time, and Rick's mom checked her watch. "Oh, look what time it is! I hope the baby wakes up soon," she said.

"It's almost the end of her naptime. I'll go in and get her now, and then I'll take you home," I said, walking into Roseanne's room.

She was still sound asleep in her crib. I reached down to pick her up. I knew the second I touched her that something was very wrong. She was warm but limp. She wouldn't wake up. Everything in my head screamed "NO!"

I quickly wrapped a blanket around Roseanne and rushed past my mother-in-law. "Something is wrong!" I shrieked in a panic. "We have to get her to the doctor right now. She's not moving. My baby is not moving!"

Shaking, I dialed the office of our pediatrician and told them what had happened. "Bring her in right now, we'll be waiting for you," said the nurse.

My mind was racing but, since I had to drive, I had to keep it together. Luckily the doctor's office was only a couple of blocks from the house. My mother-in-law held Roseanne in her arms as I clutched the steering wheel, my palms sweating. I took the baby, ran into the office and handed her to the nurse as I stood alone in the middle of the hall. My mother-in-law walked in and came up beside me.

After what seemed like an eternity the nurse came back and took us into the doctor's lounge in the back. We sat and waited in silence. *I am so calm,* I thought. *How can I be so calm?* I felt a hand on my shoulder. When I looked up I saw that it was not the first nurse who had met us at the door but Lenore, the RN. We went to high school together and had known each other for years. I was twenty-six now and she was a little older than me. Her eyes glistened with tears. The doctor stood behind her. I scanned his face for a reaction. Did he have tears in his eyes? I wasn't sure. I looked around. One whole wall in the room was covered with shelves filled with books. Some were huge and thick with rich leather bindings. Books made me feel warm, safe. I wanted to go into them, deep into their pages where no one could ever find me.

I realized that the doctor was standing beside me now. Everyone was looking at me. Everyone was quiet; too quiet. Then there was a great commotion; a huge noise. I was not sure where all the noise was coming from. Then a slow, horrible realization set in.

I spoke, "She's dead?"

"Yes," said the doctor. "Can I get you anything?" he asked.

No one was aware of all the noise in my head, just me. *"Can I get you anything? Can I get you anything? Can I get you anything?"* The question seemed to echo in my brain, to bounce back and forth. It vibrated, getting louder: *"Get you anything? Get you anything? Get you anything?"* until it felt like someone was screaming it in my ears. *"GET YOU ANYTHING!"*

There was too much noise. How could I think? Everyone was talking. Someone was even laughing. "Can I get you anything? What kind of stupid fucking question is that?"

Now someone was putting a little white pill in my hand and a glass of water in the other. My mother-in-law sat expressionless. "Pray for her," she whispered and then mentioned something about calling a pastor and my father-in-law. Someone had gotten hold of Rick and said that he was on his way.

"What the fuck for?" came a voice, "What do I need him for?

"I want to see her," I said standing up. "I want to see my daughter."

The doctor said, "No, that's not a good idea."

Suddenly there was a calm, a quiet in my head. In a strong, matter-of-fact way I announced, "She is my daughter; I am not leaving here before I see her." Was it the little white pill that gave me this sudden composure?

The doctor realized that I was not going to take no for an answer and he led me to the small, sterile examination room. Paradoxically, the room took on huge proportions, as did the examining table where my daughter lay. The room was so cold, so antiseptic. My beautiful baby, so bright, so vibrant, was surrounded by shiny, cold, steel equipment and white walls, on a piece of white paper, covered by another piece of white paper.

She was such a delicate, fragile, serious little girl, not brought to smiles easily. It wasn't that she was unhappy or that she cried a lot, she just did not give up her smiles quickly. To get an out-loud giggle took some effort. She did love music and one of her favorites was "Elvira," by The Oak Ridge Boys. She would bounce up and down when the lines "*Giddy up-ompa-ompa-mou-mou,*" would come on.

I loved to dress her up in cute little-girl outfits. She had one on today that her grandma—my mom—had made. It was a pretty pink-and-white checkered jumpsuit with a white collar and delicate lace trim, with matching white socks with pink lacey trim.

I lifted the paper and touched her cheek, stroking her fine, wispy blonde hair. Her pale blue eyes were closed, forever. I reached under the paper to find her hand. She was still warm and soft. How could she be dead? I looked up at the doctor and then at the nurse. They looked back at Roseanne. My eyes begged, *why?* There were no answers.

Life cannot end like this. Questions began to rush through my head. Heaven? What was heaven? There had to be a heaven. Life could not stop here, not like this, not here in this cold room, under a piece of paper. More questions whirled. I became aware once more of Lenore who was now guiding me out of the examining room door and back to the doctor's lounge.

Rick was there, sobbing. "No, no, not our baby!" he said. We hugged each other. We stood and just held each other. Finally, it was time to go.

The doctor said there would have to be an autopsy to find the cause of death and that the coroner would come and see us when that was determined. We left in shock, lost in our grief.

The coroner did come to see us at Rick's parents' home the next day. He concluded that Roseanne had died from sudden infant death syndrome or SIDS.

"Crib death," he said impersonally. "No one's fault, no one understands this, child just stops breathing." He handed me a pamphlet and then he was gone. The words echoed in my brain but meant nothing: *Crib death, sudden infant death syndrome, crib death.*

For the next couple days I made phone calls, made funeral arrangements, took care of all the details, took care of my family, and took care of Rick's family. I was walking efficiency. Maybe it was the little white pills the doctor had given me. People worried about my inevitable collapse. Through this whole period I felt like I was standing outside of my body, watching myself perform. I knew I had to stay strong, to manage. Now was not the time to be weak.

Occasionally a flood of sadness would overtake me and the result was a fiasco. The first occasion was when we returned to our house to find a burial outfit for Roseanne. Rick and I were in her bedroom. I already knew what I wanted her to wear so it should have been a fairly quick, in-and-out procedure. An overwhelming anger overcame me, I didn't want Rick there. "What kind of father was he? Tell him to get lost." I heard a voice—a very masculine, angry voice—in my head say, "He was away drunk all the time anyway. Don't let him be a part of this—do not dignify him in this way." I snapped. Rick had stepped out in the hall for a minute and so I locked the door and refused to let him in. I could hear him jiggling the door and calling me. After a while I began to feel calm and then the strength to manage came back. I opened the door and let Rick in and we calmly went about our solemn task.

A child's death is so horrible for everyone—not just the parents. It seemed I had to be a support to everyone around me: my parents, my sisters, everyone—or perhaps I was assuming that position. After a painful few days, all the arrangements were made and it was time for the viewing the night before the funeral. It had become very important for me to say one last farewell to Roseanne, and I wanted my family with me. The only one who protested to any extent was Dad. He did go but was so deeply affected that he couldn't stay and left the funeral home abruptly.

We had picked a beautiful pure white casket with gold handles. The interior was white satin. Rosanne looked like an angel on a cloud. She wore a favorite dress of mine. It was pale yellow organza—I had heard somewhere that yellow was a happy color—with tiny raised white velvet polka dots. She wore shiny red patent leather shoes that reminded me of the ruby slippers Dorothy wore in the *Wizard of Oz*. She held her favorite teddy bear in her arms.

I leaned down and placed a red rose beside her in the casket. Looking at my sweet angel I thought of Heaven, and a childhood memory of Great-Grandma Annie came to me. She was my dad's grandma on his mother's side and had passed away when I was fourteen. How strange to think of her now. It was a simple memory. The family was all sitting together around the table at mealtime and Great-Grandma Annie was saying grace as she always did. It was never a formal prayer but one that would include things like praise for God's love and protection, gratitude for different things, like good crops and health and family. It was different each time. Then she would end by asking for God's blessing on the food and each of the family members, and a thank-you to Jesus the Savior. My dad would often mock her while she prayed. She was deaf so luckily she didn't hear him. His favorite was, "Father, Son and Holy Ghost, whoever eats the fastest gets the most." I wished he wouldn't say those things. I loved Great-Grandma Annie and I felt bad when Dad made fun of her like that.

I wondered if Roseanne and Great-Grandma Annie were together now; if maybe there were picnics in Heaven under huge lilac trees. I hoped so. Even the thought of it gave me a sense of peace. I just could not accept that this little darling could be brought into this life and then cease to exist so quickly. There was more. There had to be more. Yes, this sweet child was now in Heaven. I was sure of it.

I cried an unending stream of tears. She was in Heaven. I was here on Earth—alone, and inconsolable.

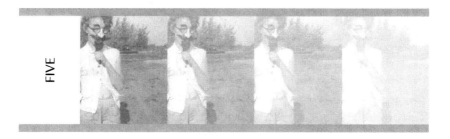

# FIVE

# Out of the Fog

The pain of Roseanne's death hung over me like a fog for a long time. I was in shock for many months and had to drag myself out of bed in the morning. She was as bright as the morning sun, and without her in my life the days were filled with darkness. With no baby to care for I slowly began to get more into the trucking business with Rick. Hard work and long hours helped fill the time and somewhat ease the agony. The business was booming at this time and my help was a definite asset.

Ironically, Rick's drinking slowed down for several months after Roseanne's death—something I had prayed for when she was alive—and our marriage strengthened during this otherwise awful time. Rick and I were both very hard workers and that leant itself to a good working relationship; it also meant we didn't have to talk much about things that were personal and painful.

Still, the memories of our baby were around every corner in our home: her scent, her laughter, her cries and the enduring loop of that horrible day when I found her lifeless in her crib. Living there without her was just too painful for both of us so decided to move. We bought a very nice but small home on the edge of town. It was on a one-acre parcel of land and had a lot of trees, both planted and wild, and a nice garden spot. It had a double-car garage, which appealed to Rick. Within a couple years Rick built a huge addition to the house giving us a large family room and another bedroom.

The trucking business, along with the remodeling of the new home and yard, demanded a lot of our time. The work was therapeutic for us, giving us goals and something to look forward to. We were able to reach a kind of calm in our relationship that we hadn't had in a long while, if ever. A few months or so after we had moved into our new home the social worker who had handled Roseanne's adoption met with us. It was a regular visit and standard for such circumstances. Toward the end of the meeting she said, "I know that Rosanne can never be replaced but there are still so many children who need loving homes. Have you considered adopting another child? While you might not feel ready just yet, the wait time to adopt a Caucasian infant is now three years so if you want to I suggest you begin the process as soon as possible."

We didn't hesitate, "Yes!" we both said in unison. She smiled and nodded in approval.

Although we had been down this road before, we would have to update the initial grueling home study along with our references. Strangely, the study never inquired about problem drinking in the home. Rick remained much better in that regard, going on a bender every once in awhile, but he certainly wasn't drunk every day the way he used to be. And so the next three years passed relatively smoothly and quickly.

One day we received a phone call out of the blue, as we had with Roseanne. "I have great news," said the social worker. "We have a baby boy for you and you can meet him in five days." It's funny how you wait for years for this then, when a baby arrives, you have to get ready immediately. It's like having too much time and not enough time all at once. The home study had been completed so the only thing left was to do was meet the child and approve of him. Apparently sometimes the chemistry just isn't there and the adoption doesn't happen. I couldn't imagine holding a three-month-old baby and not bringing him home!

When the day to see him finally arrived, Rick and I sat excitedly in the waiting room at the facility in Redman. A woman walked past us in the hallway with a baby in a yellow-and-white blanket. *Is that him,* I wondered? We waited for what seemed a very long time after that when finally the social worker brought this little person back into the room and left him with us. "Oh, look Rick," I said, "he's beautiful." I held him, so afraid he would cry, but he didn't.

Soon the social worker had come back and asked, "So what do you think? Would you like this little boy for your son?"

"Yes, of course," we both said, as I rocked him gently in my arms. "Welcome to your new family." He was a little over three months old and had already been named. We had the option of leaving it the same or changing it. We decided to rename him Craig.

I was fearful and nervous on the five-hour trip home—far more so than with Roseanne. I wanted to keep him comfortable and happy since he was now in strange surroundings. Somehow I knew it would be okay if we could just get home and he didn't cry.

The first few months at home with Craig were especially hard, not necessarily physically but emotionally. The fear of losing another child to SIDS was sometimes overwhelming. I spent hours standing by his crib making sure he was breathing. I'd often awaken in the middle of the night just to check on him.

Craig was such a dream. He was a smiling, happy baby. In fact he was so joyful that people would often ask me, "Does he ever cry?" Of course he did but not often. Thankfully this was a quiet and content time in my marriage, too. As I said, Rick's drinking had slowed down considerably anyway, but then one day he said, "I want to sober up completely and join AA. Would you support me?"

This was the answer to all my prayers and so I said, "I'm behind you 100 percent!"

Up until this time I would have a drink once in awhile but only rarely. I stopped completely to help Rick, which wasn't really an issue for me at that time because I wasn't drinking that much to begin with. These were wonderful times. We had a new lease on life, new friends; indeed it seemed a new marriage.

When Craig was about two years old, we decided it was important to go to church on a regular basis. People in the AA program and some members of Rick's family played a large part in influencing our decision, which they said would help Rick deal with the temptation of alcohol. We joined Rick's family church—he had been raised as a strong Mennonite. It was a very progressive modern church family with many young couples and young families.

This was all new to me because I had no religious upbringing and had attended church only for weddings and funerals. Immediately, however, I embraced Christianity and everything the church had to offer. I loved the feeling I got there and also, because I was an avid learner, immersed myself in reading the Bible. This church family embraced me and I soon became very active in a variety of capacities. I grew spiritually along with Craig; telling him Bible stories was my way of catching up with what I thought I had missed as a child. I reveled in the knowledge that there was a God and he loved me.

Right after we adopted Craig, we decided to once again try to adopt another child. It would be another long waiting period so if we were going down this road, we needed to make the decision immediately. Having two would be good for them both. Two children was also the maximum our provincial government would adopt to any one family. And so, three years after Craig came into our lives, we adopted Cory.

Four months old, he had chubby red cheeks, lots of dark brown hair and dark blue eyes. Rick and I noticed immediately, even on the trip home, how he constantly rotated his hands and feet, something we would find out later to be a symptom of fetal alcohol syndrome . Nothing was going to come easy for Cory. Once he was able to walk and get out of his crib I had to lay with him every night to get him to sleep; sometimes it took ten minutes, sometimes two hours. I sang to him and told him stories, the same ones every night, over and over again. Rick refused to help me with this and the lack of sleep was getting to both me and the baby. Finally my family doctor gave in and put Cory on medication; we both needed the sleep.

Craig and Cory were polar opposites. Where Craig was calm, Cory was overactive to the extreme. I realized quickly that I would have to summon completely different parenting skills with Cory than I had with Craig. I had gotten Cory a referral to a child psychologist a year or so before he started kindergarten. A series of tests revealed that he had attention deficit hyperactivity disorder and mild Tourette's Syndrome. This was all caused by fetal alcohol syndrome , now referred to as fetal alcohol spectrum disorder. There were definitely times in his life that I was angry at his biological mom, because so many, many things were so difficult for him.

I realized quickly that the anger didn't serve any useful purpose; this was the hand that we were dealt, and besides Cory had this incredible, infectious personality that endeared him to most everyone he would meet. The church family loved him and he was the center of attention for many Christmas programs. Because of his hyperactivity issues he couldn't stand still but had a great ear for music, so he always kept time even if he couldn't remember the words to the songs.

Through trial and error we did succeed in finding natural activities that seemed to calm him. He loved to fish and, much to our surprise, he would stand perfectly still when he had a fishing pole in his hand. This was such a gift, and he and his dad spent many, many hours fishing together. When he was older he and Rick would go hunting, also an activity that requires quiet and stillness, and once again this was something that captured all his energy and attention.

There seemed to be no simple formula to how his memory retrieval system worked, so the experts—child psychologists and pediatricians—kept trying different approaches. He was constantly being tested and analyzed. Some suggested medication; others no medication. We tried different diets and behavior modification. Each year he and I had a different teacher and a different tactic. To be a good parent you need to be your child's advocate; it is a full-time job, especially for a mother of a child with disabilities.

We also discovered that Cory had an extremely high pain threshold and I had to monitor him very carefully because he could hurt himself severely and not know it. One of my biggest fears was that he could not gauge temperature and so could easily suffer frostbite or worse. In Canada during wintertime this is a big issue. On the days when it got down to minus 30 degrees, I had to remind teachers at Cory's elementary school to make sure that he was not on the outdoor skating rink. He liked going out then because there were no other kids on the ice! When he had a doctor's appointment because his throat hurt for an extended period of time, the specialist was aghast at how scarred his throat was from previous infections—and yet he never complained. This is when his tonsils were removed.

The most wonderful advice I ever got on raising Cory came from an elderly lady in our church who brought up six children, mostly as a single mom. On a day when I was particularly exasperated with his behavior she looked me calmly in the eye and said, "Is this going to make any difference in five years?" It was a simple yet profound question that threw me a lifeline in trying times.

I had different rules for Cory than I did for Craig. I often wondered how Craig viewed all of this. It's much different for an adult to put things in perspective. Life had certainly changed when Cory arrived. There was no doubt about that. Life had changed for everyone. Suddenly things like sitting still in church, or finishing your supper, going to bed on time, didn't apply anymore, or didn't apply to Cory, and the consequences for his misbehavior certainly must have seemed very unfair. Cory was three years younger and had spent two years in kindergarten so I was able to keep their activities quite separate for the most part, but for some of Cory's younger years, especially when I was also so busy with so many other things, he exhausted me at home. The boys really had nothing in common; Cory was rough and tumble, sometimes out of control, and sometimes mean to Craig. It became apparent that the easiest way to manage the situation was to keep them separate.

Through all of this, the church provided me with a physical

and emotional sanctuary. It had a wonderful children's outreach program for elementary-school aged kids that started in September and ran until April, meeting once a week. It was jam-packed with wonderful things that kids like: hayrides, sleepovers, and movie and pizza nights. It also incorporated what was called a Pal Program that involved matching each child up with an adult in the church, sort of a "big brother/big sister" idea with a Christian emphasis.

The year Craig was old enough to join the program I became its coordinator and stayed in this position until Cory quit going. I loved it. At its peak we drew nearly seventy children—an all-time record. Sometimes more than half were from families outside of the church. This was what a good part of the program was all about: sharing the Gospel with the community. I was like a kid, new in her faith. I was growing up spiritually with my boys, especially Craig. The Bible stories I taught him were new to me as well and I learned along with him. The market was full of great products to teach kids the Gospel. I loved to incorporate them into the club's programming. It was fun and fresh and it gave me a real sense of purpose. If someone had a talent, I found a way to get them involved. It was an exciting place to be on Tuesdays, in fact so much so that parents started to show up early to have coffee in the kitchen, coming to visit before picking up their kids. Some of those parents ended up at my own kitchen table, giving their lives to Christ and becoming members of the church family.

These were good times. After so much grief and heartache with Rick's alcoholism, the loss of Roseanne and our struggles with Cory, things seemed to be going well and life was wonderful.

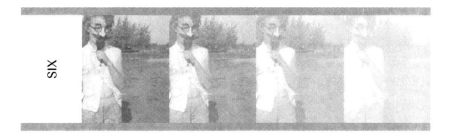

SIX

# *Last Call for Redemption*

My dad had been diagnosed with lung cancer just prior to our moving our family to the farm I grew up on as a child. It was terminal and aggressive, spreading rapidly. About a month after his diagnosis, we had to maintain a twenty-four hour vigil of sitting with him early on, not because death was imminent but because he had refused to quit smoking. He could not be left alone because he had become a safety risk, constantly falling asleep with a lit cigarette.

My mother, my sisters and I set up rotating schedule ensuring that he was never unattended. The erratic shifts left me feeling like I had chronic jet lag and the circumstances were very stressful. I still had the children to attend to and was trying to work on fixing up our house. This ordeal would have taken its toll on the stoutest of hearts and minds—we did this for almost five months—so I attributed my mood swings, depression and even the night episodes on this turn of events.

I was very involved with the church at this time and was grateful for the community support I got from them. My spiritual metamorphosis did bring with it an enormous feeling of responsibility, however, for the lost souls in my family, chiefly my father. As his death grew imminent, I felt compelled to get him to repent for all his sins before he died. His abuse of prescription pain pills for his arthritis and over-the-counter medication, combined with alcohol, had escalated to an all-out addiction. I don't think the local doctor even considered him an alcoholic—just a social drinker. That was "normal" in the place and time in which we lived but certainly would have been different today. My parents' relationship was never good, but this made it completely disintegrate. He never became physically violent with Mom, but was constantly emotionally abusive, playing all kinds of mind games. They fought constantly and my mother looked miserable most of the time. If only Dad would repent, I could relax and let him go; knowing he would not burn in Hell, all would be fine. Our whole church prayed for his salvation, which only heaped more pressure on me.

I had to help my dad. That is what dutiful daughters do. I lost track of how many times I heard Dad tell me how important it was to be a "good girl." Good girl aside, there were so many times while caring for him in his final days, that I would think, *I am so glad he is dying.* Was it the stress of sleeplessness? I don't know, but of course I always felt guilty. I would jolt out of this and replace it with: *How can you say this about your own father? And you call yourself a Christian?* But the feelings kept coming nonetheless. I would be absolutely elated that he was about to die. I would then fall on my knees in prayer, "Please God, forgive me for such a vile thought!"

I knew how much God loved me. Still, it was a time of confusion. I was coming to terms with all I had been told about God's abundant love—but I had questions. Ted Bundy had been executed and while on death row had declared himself a Christian, forgiven of his serial killings. Is it possible, can someone as horrific as that be in Heaven? Would I share Heaven with someone like that someday? Of course, God's love was that big, that all encompassing. I knew that. I sat down and wrote my dad a letter. I told him there was nothing God couldn't forgive, nothing out of God's reach. I was so careful in my explanation—all I wanted was for him to understand how simple it was.

But time was running out. He was in the hospital now and conscious less and less. My time by his bed was spent praying to keep Dad out of Hell. Finally, two days before he died, he called Rick and me to his bedside, something he had never done before. Though fragile he looked directly into my eyes and said. "Don't worry, I am ready to go."

I wept with relief. I took it as a sign that my prayers were answered. His soul had been "saved." Dad had surrendered to God. I had done my part.

Three weeks after Dad's funeral I sat in my car outside the cemetery gates. Maybe it was my grief, but I couldn't remember driving there. The motor was running. I sat staring out at the grounds, covered under a foot of snow. "How did I get here? Why am I here?" I said out loud, completely confused. I finally got out of the car and made my way through the snowdrifts to Dad's grave. Suddenly in a voice I didn't recognize, with a laugh not my own, I threw my head back and started to laugh hysterically. The urge to dance overwhelmed me so there I was, arms in the air, my feet moving as best as they could in the deep snow, dancing between the tombstones like I was at a disco.

"I'm glad, I'm glad, I'm glad, glad, glad! I hate you, hate you, *hate* you!" I sang and laughed while kicking snow into the air. "I'm happy you're dead! Happy, happy, *happy!*"

Then it hit me like a ton of bricks: I realized where I was and what I was doing. I ran back to the car, stumbling and falling in the snow several times, screaming and crying, tears streaming down my face.

I got back to my car and sat behind the wheel for several minutes trying to get my breath. This was unbelievable! This was insanity! Who would do such a thing? I looked around to make sure no one was watching. No one must ever know about this. Waves of guilt ran over me. What kind of daughter was I? What kind of Christian? I was shaking and nauseous.

I closed my eyes and tried to recall an image of my father's face so I could tell him how truly sorry I was for this terrible act I had just committed. But instead I could only pull memories of how his life had spiraled out of control in the last couple of years. With my newfound Christianity, I had worked very hard at trying to get Dad to quit drinking, especially after seeing the wonderfully positive changes in my husband's life when he had stopped. But I had learned a lot about addictions through the Twelve-Step programs and knew you really couldn't force anyone to sober up: they had to make that decision themselves. As much as I knew that to be true, I had continued to try and with every failed attempt I resented him more, which I immediately followed with a load of self-induced guilt. A "good" daughter should be able to help her father. And for sure, a good daughter shouldn't feel the way I just had about her dad.

I stayed away from the cemetery as much as possible after that.

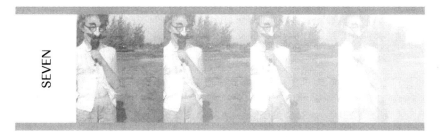

# SEVEN

# The Shadow in the Light

Rick and I had thrown ourselves into developing the farmstead. I especially loved the huge garden we'd planted. I tended it with pride, showing it off to all who visited. Rick had even built me a greenhouse, so I started all my own bedding plants. They were so abundant that I gave many trays away to neighbors.

I spent hours cheerfully cleaning up debris, dead grass and trees. We worked tirelessly repairing things and building a handsome ranch-style fence to separate the barnyard from the main yard where our house and garden sat. I had a huge strawberry and raspberry patch that I bordered with an assortment of colorful flowers. The kids loved the snapdragons and used them in flower puppet shows. Delphiniums grew blue spikes over three feet tall. Towering over everything were sunflowers, which grew to heights of fourteen feet. We harvested tomatoes for jars of homemade soup, juice, salsa and pizza sauce.

The boys loved to hide in the lush garden growth, eating raw peas and carrots—as well as using them as ammunition in their robust game of cops and robbers. Craig and Cory happily roamed the yard, climbed the trees, caught frogs, and played with the dog, the many cats and bunnies, and the six baby goats. They helped tend the chickens and imitated them with their bobbing heads. Rick decided to raise some feeder cattle so the big barn and existing fences were put to good use. The whole community complimented us on the improvements. Life was great.

That's why I was completely perplexed by the strange, haunting feelings I was having; like someone was watching my every move. It would creep up on me out of nowhere. The occasional night terrors didn't stop and more than once I found myself wide awake in the pre-dawn hours, clutching my pillow in fear. No amount of hard work, fresh-cut flowers on my kitchen counter, or happy family activities could shake the sensation of doom that gripped me.

Then came the flashing snapshots of bizarre experiences. The first one hit on a hot August day. I was looking out my kitchen window, which faced the barnyard. The boys were playing with a new little goat that had been born that spring. They were chasing each other and the kid back and forth around the pen where the mother goat was tethered. They were giggling. I could hear them from the house. They were having so much fun that I decided to join them.

I started toward them and as I did, I glanced to my right. I wasn't even sure why I did that. This was the north side of the yard. The thick natural growth of trees that had always been there was full and lush as always. When I lived here as a child this was where the family outhouse had been. I paused for a second—and then I saw the vision of a man, blocking the sunlight, his cap hanging slightly sideways, pants around his ankles. I felt like I had been kicked in the stomach, I gasped for air stumbling backward. I thought I was going to black out; I had to get back into the house now, quickly. He wasn't really there, it was like the flash of a movie projector image—but the fear that it brought was terrifyingly real.

Back in the house I worked to regain my composure. Coffee, black strong coffee, that's what I needed. I filled the decanter with water, and added enough grounds to make a strong pot. "Breathe," I said to myself, "just breathe."

The fear passed as quickly as it had come and my thoughts

returned back to my children playing. Sitting at my kitchen table, I looked out the south window and again my mind filled with the beauty outside: The profusion of flowers that I had planted set against 160 acres of golden yellow canola in full bloom; the backdrop of the majestic blue Pasquia Hills; the swaying row of rich green maple trees that the boys loved to climb. I lifted the coffee cup to my lips and was surprised to see that my hands were shaking. It seemed odd that my body was so stressed out when my mind seemed so serene. I thought to myself, *Rick is happy here. Craig and Cory are happy here. Am I happy here? I think I am. Then why am I shaking? Is there no satisfaction in any of this? What is wrong with me?*

These feelings churned around in my mind: feelings of anxiety that I was really *not* happy, and guilt because my children and husband clearly loved it here. And wasn't that what mattered most—the family? Besides, coming here was as much my idea as anyone's.

Then gloom struck: "I'm *not* happy here," I said out loud. "In fact I *hate* it!" It was something about the yard that upset me; the house was the only place I felt any sense of serenity. Even with the night terrors, the house held peace for me during the day. It was so confusing. I could also spend time in the garden, which was in the front yard, but the back yard held this horrible grip on me. The boys were coming in now. I forced myself to put on a happy face. I could not let them see me like this—again.

I had not told anyone about the night terrors, but the strain of them, my increasing bouts of depression, mood swings, and crying was making my family worried and tense. I didn't want to be that kind of mother—these were my children and I loved them so much.

There had to be a logical reason for this and therefore a logical solution. Perhaps it was a hormonal one. My monthly periods were getting increasingly painful to the point that the cramps were almost unbearable.

I set up an appointment with my family physician, entirely convinced that this must be the case. I never mentioned the feelings of foreboding, seeing the naked man or the night terrors: that would just be way too weird. I concentrated on the mood swings and the horrible monthly pain.

My doctor found problems with my uterus and fibroids on one ovary and suggested a partial hysterectomy. Another woman might have cringed at such a diagnosis but I was delighted. Surely this was the reason for all my problems and hopefully the surgery would end my misery.

The surgery did provide relief from the monthly misery of my period. Being pain free was pure joy. I had renewed energy and was downright euphoric—but not for long. A few months later I was driving home from town; nothing out of the ordinary. The boys were both in school and I had run errands and gone shopping in the afternoon. I was listening to a local country-and-western station on the car radio, tapping my fingers on the steering wheel to the song "On the Wings of a Dove" by Ferlin Husky. It's an old country classic. I had heard my dad, accompanied by Grandpa and Grandma, play it many times when I was a kid.

Suddenly a severe pain, like a hot knife, ran through my uterus. I screamed and slammed on the brakes. Oddly, the pain was gone as quickly as it had come. I turned off the radio and sat in silence, trying to figure out what had just happened. Then it hit me: a strange, strong smell in the car. It was the odor of sweat, heavy and thick, the way a man smells after a long hard day's work. It was him, the vision I had seen in our yard, the man with the cap on slightly sideways, in the doorway, blocking out the sun. I drove home, shaking the entire way.

The operation had not been the answer. I cried out, "God, please, what is happening to me? Help me! You promised that if I followed you my life would be filled with love and light! Don't leave me here in the darkness!"

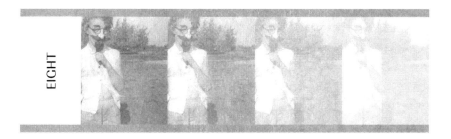

# EIGHT

# Feeling Like a Fraud

I had always liked the pastor of my church, Pastor Paul. He is a wonderful, compassionate and kind man. At the time he was in his mid sixties, married with grown children. We hit it off immediately. On my way out of my first service at his parish he smiled and hugged me, saying, "Oh, it's so nice to hug someone who isn't a fence post."

Chuckling, I replied, "Yes, well, there is way too much padding here to be a fence post!" We both had a good laugh and the tone was set for our relationship.

When the hysterectomy failed to solve my problems I decided to call the pastor for a counseling session. I was completely at my wit's end and I trusted him implicitly. I told him, "I've got two beautiful children and a husband who loves me. "I should be happy but most days I'm very depressed, like something is out to get me. Maybe if I pray more," I said, "Maybe Jesus will lift this veil of impending doom I feel." As comfortable as I was with him, I still could not bring myself to reveal the other bizarre things that were occurring.

"Sounds like depression to me," he said. I nodded my head, hoping that maybe there was still a way out from this.

The counseling sessions with Pastor Paul were comforting but it was only a temporary relief. We talked about so many issues— raising children, being a Christian wife, my role in the church—then every session would end in prayer and I would be momentarily better. But on the way home I would start to feel uneasy, and the closer I got to the farm the worse it would get. Eventually I quit seeing Pastor Paul because the comfort he offered at his office seemed to make how I felt at home worse. It was like going from an air-conditioned room out into the desert in the summer. It almost seemed better to feel moderately bad all the time than to intersperse periods of sweet relief in a sea of abject misery. Instead of finding a spiritual solution to my problems my confusion deepened.

The harder I tried to make the confusion, the paranoia, the visions, the night terrors go away the more the internal struggle intensified. I began to think there was more going on here than a woman losing her mind. Bible studies, church involvement, all the happiness that the Christian life was supposed to provide seemed to be slipping further and further from my grasp. Bearing this burden alone, in secrecy, was nearly intolerable. But how could I possibly reveal all the details of this to anyone? I lived in a small community and people would think I was crazy. My family would be made to carry that burden and I could not do that to them.

While I was falling apart inside, from the outside people thought I was a model citizen. I was everything the Christian wife and mother should be. I was encouraged again and again to lead the women's Bible study group. The children's program had been so successful and so inviting that moms gathered often not just for their children but for themselves. It had become a place for them to come together and to seek out my advice and to pray for them. Ironically, my popularity and leadership status both with the kids and their parents was blossoming at exactly the same time I was spiraling downward. I felt like a total fraud. If they knew the truth about me they wouldn't want to be anywhere near me.

"All this work, all this activity that I'm doing with bubbling enthusiasm, is a joke, a complete farce," I said to myself. "Is this a big game of pretend for everyone?"

Meanwhile, back on the acreage, Rick had purchased more goats. In order to keep them out of the front yard, he decided to put a fence along the row of trees that ran along the north side of the property. When my parents owned the land, this had been the place where the outhouse had been. The chicken coop and a chop bin had also been close by. Those old buildings had long since been demolished and except for extra thick green growth from the rich deposits of manure, there was no other evidence that they had ever existed.

Building the fence was a big job for one person so I offered to give Rick a hand as he dug fence postholes with the tractor. We had been out there for some time when it hit: the same ferocious pain that leveled me in the car. It was like someone had stabbed me with a knife deep in my vagina. I doubled over in agony, falling to the ground and holding my abdomen. I saw the vision of the man again, tall and with his pants down around his ankles. This time I saw a small boy and a small girl; the boy on his hands and knees in the grass, the little girl crouched against a granary. There was also a black-and-white dog. Then the vision was gone.

It left as quickly as it had appeared. I slumped against the tractor. My whole body shook. I felt the sobs coming again. My husband came from around the other side of the tractor. "What's wrong? Are you all right?" he asked.

"No!" I cried. "I have to go to the house right now!"

I all but ran inside, the pain still searing through my uterus.

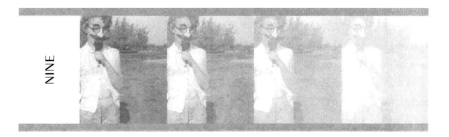

NINE

# *Unfaithful*

Surely I was going insane. I made an appointment with my family doctor. I didn't like the sad, confused feeling I was experiencing. "I've been going through a rough time," I explained, "and I just can't get any rest." With that, he wrote up a prescription for me, the same as he had to help me cope with Roseanne's death. Medication was not my first choice but the tranquillizers calmed me somewhat and helped me sleep. This in turn allowed me to get the boys off to school in the morning, hold a part-time job as a home-health aide during the day, and keep up my church responsibilities. Although I could function I was still emotionally exhausted.

Tension between Rick and me was mounting daily. He was tremendously overworked as was I. We were both stretched to the limit. The worse our problems got, the more his sexual requirements increased. In fact, he was so dissatisfied with our sex life that he set up a meeting with the associate pastor to discuss it. This hurt me tremendously. I thought I was being a good wife, now I was told—*not so.* "A man needs his sex," said the associate pastor.

I rebutted with, "A woman needs some communication, some appreciation." We saw him a number of times and thought we were making progress until we learned that his wife was discovered having an affair with another married member of the congregation. We decided he may not be such a good couples' therapist after all!

Adding fuel to the fire were our mounting financial problems. We had taken on too much. We were trying to raise livestock, which neither of us really had the experience to do, so we made many wrong, costly decisions: we took out huge operating loans, bought expensive feed, and so many small things. We really didn't see, or perhaps want to see, that we were slowly drowning financially. My escape was my part-time job. I loved taking care of others. It also gave me my own money so I could make sure nothing had to change as far as the children were concerned. Still, it was just a drop in the bucket compared to the sea of red ink that defined our family finances. This was no time for me to be falling apart. I had to buck up, be the supportive wife. Willpower and optimism aside, it was soon obvious that the only way out of our financial situation was to declare bankruptcy. This stressed me out to no end. What would we do? Could we lose our home? Could my husband find another job? What would people think? On and on it went, along with everything else I was already coping with—the night terrors, my husband not being happy with our sex life, the horrible visions in the yard. Everything was spiraling out of control.

Eventually we did declare bankruptcy. Soon Rick was enrolled in a pre-employment welding program in a city two hours away. This paid a sufficient wage to support our family and Rick soon settled nicely into the routine of being away all week and only home for the weekends, leaving me alone to look after the farm and the two young boys.

One weekend when he was home, we made an appointment with the municipal government on Monday to discuss outstanding taxes, another one of many humiliating conversations necessary in bankruptcy proceedings. While we had hoped that the bankruptcy would shield us from paying this sizeable amount of money, the meeting dashed our hopes when we discovered it would not. As the old saying goes, "There are only two things you can count on in life: death and taxes." We were able to draw up an appropriate payment plan, which meant tightening our already meager purse strings. But we committed to making it work and getting back on track financially.

Rick left for school immediately after the meeting and I returned home. Not long after I'd walked in the door I received a call from a municipal official telling me they had made a huge mistake in their calculations and that the amount we owed was very much less than what they had quoted. I was delighted with the news and wanted to share it with Rick as soon as I could.

I waited until suppertime to make sure he was home from classes. I called but he wasn't in. He was living in a boarding house, which had a main house phone. The landlady said she would give him the message as soon as he arrived. It wasn't unusual for Rick to be a little late. I knew he wasn't all that fond of the landlady's cooking, so I just assumed that maybe he went out for a burger instead.

When I didn't hear anything an hour later, I called back. "No, Mrs. Ducommun, he hasn't come in yet," said the landlady politely. When I still hadn't heard in another hour, I called again—and every hour after that for many hours.

"Mrs. Ducommun, it is now 11:00 PM and I am going to bed," the landlady's tone was definitely not cordial anymore. "I will tape a note on your husband's door so that he will be sure to see it." I had a sick feeling in the pit of my stomach and I slept very little that night.

I dialed him again at seven o'clock the next morning. The landlady said, "Yes, he just arrived and he seems pretty happy."

I was decidedly unhappy. "May I talk to him?" I asked, and I could hear her pass the phone to Rick. Shaking with anger I said, "Are you drinking again? Where were you last night?"

"Yes, I've been drinking," he said and started to cry. "I have been drinking and I have been unfaithful." Now he was sobbing.

Drinking and unfaithful; the words sat in my brain like a stone. Unfaithful. "Come home," I said, and hung up.

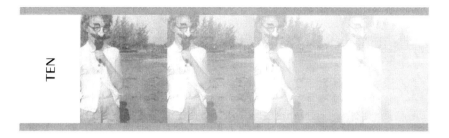

TEN

# *Searching for Peace*

"Infidelity. Infidelity!" I shouted. I was a Christian and everything in my head screamed, "this is wrong!" It was biblically and morally wrong. As I sat waiting for Rick to come home, I ran though my head various conflicting scenarios of what I would say and how I would say it:

"You have forsaken our marriage vows and betrayed our family and the church. Please leave;

"You did this because I have not been good enough in the bedroom. Let's go make love right now;

"Something is wrong and has been for a long time. Let's sit down and have a serious talk about this;

"I can't stand the sight of you. Get your things and leave this house now!"

It was so confusing, but the strongest voice ruled the day and it was talking to me and giving me directions: "Be strong. Confront him. You don't deserve any of this, so don't take it. He is shit, unworthy of you—quit pretending and get rid of him!"

Another quieter, more comforting voice said, *"It will be fine, remember your faith."*

Then someone strong said, "Don't let this take you down, you are smarter than he will ever be. Remember the welfare of the children."

I could hear them all—a cacophony of voices: some angry, some sad, and some comforting. They left me bereft and exhausted. Not that they were done with me. I had heard the voices before, for years; in fact I couldn't remember a time when they weren't there. They generally did not all talk at once. Ordinarily, it was like someone adding a suggestion or offering an observation. Occasionally, if something upsetting was going on, it would become noisier. Those times scared me. I would become fearful of how things might happen during those noisy times when there seemed to be serious disagreements.

My husband walked in the door looking like a truck had hit him. *Why is he looking so whipped?* I thought. I was the polar opposite: in control and as cool as a cucumber. Before he could utter the first word I turned to him calmly and said, "This is unforgivable."

"I just couldn't stand the loneliness, Chris, without you and the boys," he confessed. "So I started drinking again, and the women followed." So now I also knew there had been more than one. He was a beaten, pathetic man who had found solace in sex—and now he expected to get his wife and family back?

"I am going to call Pastor Paul right now," I said, and set up a meeting for that very day.

The pastor walked us through all the necessary Christian hoops: The children were too young and needed to be kept out of this; and, of course, the Christian family needed to survive above all else.

"I am so sorry. I am completely responsible for this mess and the hurt I have caused you," Rick said remorsefully. "Please give me a second chance. I won't do this again."

There were voices yelling at me inside my head, "Don't trust him! He's a liar!" and I'd silently yell back, "Go away! I want peace; peace for me and peace for my boys! Leave me alone!"

With our pastor's guidance we committed ourselves to each

other and to the Lord, and stuffed all the rest. We had only visited him a couple of times when on the way home we agreed to recommit ourselves and our marriage to God and to start a new life. I truly, deeply, forgave him and was sure life from there would work.

Rick only had a couple weeks before he would be finished with his welding course, so he went back to do that. When he got home he quickly landed a job with a local welding shop. We had been able to keep our home and so life began to slip into a comfortable routine. For the most part our relationship seemed fine. Occasionally, I would find myself suspicious and doubting him but I wanted harmony in our home so I pushed those feelings aside. With God's power I was sure we could make this work. However as more time passed the security that I had felt began to erode. I found myself doing the "kiss and sniff test" when he got home later than usual to see if I could smell any alcohol.

Before long the dialogue in my head was like a constant chatter, erratic and disjointed. A voice said, "There is *no* God! You can't trust these people!"

Another calm voice said, "Trust in God. He is your guiding light through the darkness."

Yet another said, "Just don't do anything to hurt the boys!"

There was so much noise, so much confusion; it made me feel absolutely insane. Then a small and seemingly insignificant thing forced me to look at how my behavior was affecting my children.

I had made chili for supper one night. It was a family favorite and I wanted to do something special for them. I called out the door to the boys, "Supper's ready!"

They came running to the house. "Yay, we're starving!" They washed their hands then sat down expectantly as I started ladling the chili into their bowls.

"Chili? Yuck!" moaned Cory as he scrunched up his face in disgust.

It was just a young child's response. He usually liked chili but kids' tastes change frequently and maybe he had his heart on something else. I understood this, and yet it was overwhelming. I viewed this as a personal attack. I somehow didn't have the reasoning capacity to see it for what it really was.

"You love chili! What do you mean, 'Yuck, chili?' No dinner for you. Leave the table. Go to your room! Maybe you will be hungry enough to eat chili in the morning. Leave. NOW!" I was screaming at the top of my lungs.

Craig just stared at his bowl and then quietly ate his chili. Maybe because of his calm, it didn't take but a moment for overwhelming guilt and shame to set in. How could I have screamed at my son like that?

I walked to the stairway and saw Cory standing at the top of the stairs, looking so defeated, and crying. "I'm sorry, Cory. Come down and have some chili. Please. Come back to the table," I said, near tears myself. He shook his head "no," and walked back to his bedroom.

I cringed and felt my stomach churn. I made up a fresh, hot bowl of chili and a nice thick slice of bread and took it to him. I told him again that I was sorry I had yelled at him. He was quiet but ate his chili and bread. I went to my bedroom, grabbed a pillow and screamed into it so that the boys could not hear me. How could I be so mean to my son? I collapsed on the bed and cried and cried until I finally fell asleep. I awoke an hour later to hear the boys out in the garden. I was so relieved they were okay and even having fun.

The next day I woke up to get the boys ready to catch the school bus into town. I made them French toast, exactly the way they liked it, and allowed them extra syrup. The moment they left for school, I called my doctor, completely distraught. Dr. Cooper agreed to see me that morning even though I was over thirty miles away. We had a good doctor/patient relationship; she had been through a lot with me in the past ten years and she was very understanding about seeing me at the earliest possible moment.

I sat in the examination room, crying, when the doctor walked in. "What is going on?" Dr. Cooper asked.

"I don't know, I am so scared, I am yelling at my kids over nothing," I told her.

She asked, "Tell me what you are feeling."

"I am afraid. I don't know how to control this, please help me," I said.

She asked about other behaviors, "Do you gamble? Are you a compulsive shopper? Do you eat to feel better?" By my weight I was obviously overeating—a common obsession shared by most of my family.

I was so confused I didn't know how to answer.

"I'm quite concerned about you and don't think this is a physical problem. I suggest that you see a psychiatrist. I know a good one, Dr. Baker, who visits this area once a week."

I nodded my head in agreement. Could Dr. Baker be my lifeline to sanity? I hoped so, for my sake and that of my family.

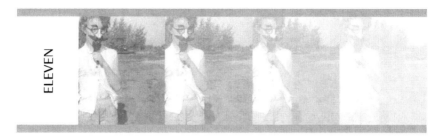

# ELEVEN

# The Missing Pieces

I began my sessions with the psychiatrist, Dr. Baker. "Dr. Cooper tells me you've been having some problems, tell me about them Mrs. Ducommun," he asked.

"I have these times when I just can't stop crying. I want to stop but I can't. It's like a faucet I can't turn off. And I'm so moody. I yell at my children for no good reason."

"Does this come with your monthly cycle?" he asked.

"I had a hysterectomy so I don't have a monthly cycle anymore. I thought that would solve the problem but it has just gotten worse," I answered.

"Has something in your life changed recently that might have brought this on?" he inquired.

"We were having some financial problems and I recently discovered that my husband was unfaithful." He nodded and scribbled on his notepad. I continued, "That was a big shock, but we've been in counseling with our pastor and things have gotten better that way."

Saying things had gotten better in my marriage was stretching the truth. After Rick's affair I never felt like anything was right again. Sometimes, because I knew sex was so important to him, I would try different sensual things to fulfill him. I really did want to please him but it was a one-way street. Rick would *never* ask what pleased me.

"Is there anything else?" Dr. Cooper asked. Yes, of course there was quite a bit more to tell but I just couldn't talk about the strange night terrors and the fragmented flashbacks I was having, even with him.

"No that is it. Just these horrible mood swings and the crying. I hope you can help me doctor. I just want peace, please, for the sake of my family."

"This sounds like a classic case of clinical depression," he answered. "I'd like to see you once a week at first. I'm going to give you some homework. I'd like you to chart your moods so that we can better pinpoint what might bring on the crying spells. In the meantime, I'm going to give you a prescription to fill. We'll try this medication and see if it helps. We can alter the dosage if we need to." I thanked him and tucked the prescription into my purse.

This began a useless year of charting moods, ten-minute meetings once a month, and trying various mood-altering medications. My moods *were* altered; I suppose I wasn't so "on edge." I was calmer and less anxious, but nothing changed the night terrors, the flashbacks or the crying.

Twelve months later I was still crying in the bathroom or into my pillow and still having night terrors. I rarely went into the back yard because of what I might see or feel. Most days it seemed like the only thing keeping me from dropping into insanity was a thread of hope that I clung to for the sake of my boys.

I was determined to make my sons' lives good ones. They so deserved it. They did not ask to be adopted by a mother who would just mentally "check out" on them. I fought tooth and nail to keep the mood swings from them, and the crying as well. I'd take them away from the farm as much as possible. We'd go fishing and have wonderful picnics. I took them to swimming lessons and on visits with their grandma. I loved these times away from the farm. I always felt like a veil had been lifted; I surmised because

I was out of the house and active. At any rate I wanted Craig and Cory to remember their childhood as fun and happy.

*Strange,* would *they remember?* I asked myself. I sure couldn't remember my younger years. Anything before I turned eleven was almost non-existent. I couldn't recall special occasions like birthday parties—or even holidays like Christmas. I worked so hard at making these times special for my sons but I had no recollection to draw from—none whatsoever.

On one of Cory's birthdays he brought four friends home after school on the bus. I filled the entire living room with balloons. Their eyes were as wide as saucers when they walked through the front door and their eyes lit up like Christmas trees when I handed each of them a tack and said, "Now go pop them all—just be careful!" They went on a balloon-popping frenzy, laughing and screaming until they were all finished. Would he remember this?

I kept trying to remember something—anything. I knew this wasn't right. It wasn't normal not to have *any* childhood memories. I came to this conclusion by nonchalantly asking my friends about their growing-up years. Several of them could recall in great detail memories from very young years—as young as age three and four. I couldn't even remember who my elementary school teachers were until grade five.

I was desperate. I began reading everything I could get my hands on as far as mental illness. I watched every talk show on depression, bought self-help books and read them cover to cover. If I believed what I read, then there was the possibility of sexual abuse in my past. But there were no memories of it. Surely I would remember something as awful as that happening to me.

The exercise of trying to piece together my past gripped me. The more I tried to solve this puzzle, the more I realized there were pieces missing. But why? Why couldn't I remember my childhood?

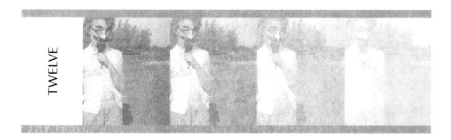

# TWELVE

# Talk Therapy

After all my research, I came to the conclusion that I needed "talk therapy" not mood-altering medications. I was also hoping I could find someone who could help me with my memory loss and provide a plan for how I might get it back. With new resolve, I searched for a counselor. There was a Christian counseling agency based in a community an hour or so from me. I hoped that the distance would help preserve my anonymity. People saw us as the perfect Christian family. I certainly didn't want to shatter that image—which I was sure would happen if anyone knew I was seeking help for mental health problems as serious as what I assumed mine to be.

I was as nervous as I'd ever been for this appointment. I had so long sought a reason for my behavior but deep down maybe I really didn't want to know. I fidgeted in the waiting room, flipping through the pages of a magazine just to give my hands something to do. A pretty, young petite brunette woman opened the door of the waiting room. "Mrs. Ducommun?" she said, extending her hand to me. "Good morning! I'm Lynette Bushman." Her appearance and perkiness caught me off guard; I'd been expecting a matronly, graying somewhat stout woman. I tried to hide my surprise and followed her into her office.

"So what brings you to our center today?" she asked.

"I've been having terrible mood swings and crying episodes for years," I answered. "I've been to my family doctor, who could not help, and he sent me to a psychiatrist for the last year. He gave me anti-depressants but that did not help either. So I've tried to find out what is wrong with me on my own. Some of the books I've been reading, well, I was thinking maybe I was sexually abused as a child." I continued, nearly out of breath, "I'm giving myself two to three weeks to fix this. I've got children to raise and I need to get on with my life."

The counselor chuckled but not in a sarcastic way. "Mrs. Ducommun, we'll need to explore why you think this happened to you and, if it did, it is going to take longer than a few weeks. But don't worry; I will be here with you every step of the way."

And so began four years of treatment with Lynette Bushman. Both she and I would refer back to that comment of fixing myself in less than a month every now and then, finding it amusing. Any apprehension that I had about her being too young or not matronly enough quickly melted away. I trusted her almost immediately and soon the beginning of a very long journey to healing got underway.

A sense of optimism infused me with a passion to attack this problem. There would be no more holding back. I was going to find out what was wrong with me. I had confided that I could not recall my early childhood years so Lynette asked me to reconstruct a picture of my life, beginning as a child, with anything concrete I had from that time.

I decided to go through pictures and anything else I had from that time to try and spark *any* kind of memory. I meticulously poured through each year of my elementary school report cards, reading comments from teachers whose faces I desperately tried to recall and couldn't, trying to spark some memory. I would read them again and again, hoping that the repetition would somehow ingrain them into my memory and become my past. I'd ask myself questions like, "What kind of student had I been? Was I good in sports? Was I popular? Did the teachers like me? Did I like school?"

I got out pictures of myself as a young girl. Oddly, looking at myself was like looking at a stranger. If my mother had not scribbled my name on the back of the photo I would not have known it was me. I thought I had always been fat. These pictures were not of a fat girl. I stared for hours at these pictures. They were typical pictures, many of which you could probably find in anyone's family photo album: Christmastime gatherings with relatives seated at the table filled with food; Great-Grandma Annie holding a child or two on her lap; birthday parties and other celebrations; the proud display of a new baby sister. Then there were glimpses of life on a farm: the arrival of a new piece of farm equipment; a harvest meal behind a combine in a wheat field; spring calves, kittens and puppies. Yet this whole collection of Norman Rockwell-esque scenes still could not spark a memory in me—none whatsoever. They were pictures of someone else's life.

Lynette didn't have much to work with so we discussed a couple of disturbing memories I *could* recall. They were in grade four. This seemed like when my memories did start, as though I had been born then. "I remember going into a cubicle in the girl's bathroom at school," I said. No one was in there, so I put some of the powdered soap from the dispenser in my hand and went into the stall to eat it."

"Do you know why you did that?" she inquired.

"I'm not sure. I wanted to make myself get sick; maybe so that I wouldn't have to participate in the singing competition? Really, I don't know," I said shaking my head.

"I also remember this wooden jewelry box I had in my room. I hit myself on the forehead with it, over and over again. It left this horrible black and blue lump. When my parents asked me about it I told them I got into a fistfight at school. Why would I do that?"

As strange as these things were the most disturbing memory was going shopping with my mother for a pair of sneakers. I recounted this episode to Lynette: "It was the end of summer, just before the start of school, and I needed new shoes. We found a pair in the local Robinsons department store. They were pale blue with white laces.

I loved them. The salesperson brought out few boxes with slightly different sizes, then left to go help another customer. 'Here, Chris, try these on first,' said my mom. No one had tried on these shoes yet and the laces were only put through the first set of holes. I took the balled-up laces out of the shoes. *Now what do I do?* I thought. *How do you lace up the shoes?* I had no earthly idea. I was going into grade five, I should know how. I started to try, but nothing made sense. With each failed attempt it felt like someone was squeezing my stomach. I heard someone laughing and making fun of me. I wanted to run away and hide. My mom didn't see any of this, she was at the cashier's till talking to a lady she apparently knew.

"Mom would be angry that I had done nothing. She needed to get home and start supper. There was that laughter again. Where was it coming from? There was no one else around. I didn't understand. *Oh no, Mom is walking this way, I must get the shoes laced up.*

"'What are you doing?' Mom asked.

"'I don't know how,' I replied in a little girl's voice.

"'What do you mean?' Mom snapped.

"'I don't know how!' I whimpered.

"'Oh I don't have time for this,' she said, irritated. She grabbed the shoes, laced them, and handed them back to me. I put them on and, shamefaced, stuffed the ends of the laces in the sides. I did not know how to tie them. I had been tying my own laces since I was five years old—one of the first skills they teach you in school so the teacher isn't constantly bending over. The girl in the Robinson store, apparently me, did not know how, she had not been taught—and she didn't know why."

I expected Lynette to laugh but she did not and I was grateful. I was feeling quite comfortable with her and a trust was developing. I didn't hide things from her as I had done with the other doctors. I would always share any new memories or discoveries with her. Oddly, though, I began to have blackouts about my counseling sessions. It was like the amnesia about the past was rubbing off on the present. Sometimes I could just not remember my time spent with Lynette.

It also happened away from the therapist's office. One day I found a black-and-white picture of myself, definitely pre-school, I looked to be about four years old. It was pinned to the bulletin board beside my kitchen phone. I had no idea how it got there—but it could only have been placed there by me. I shared this with Lynette and also told her about my inability to remember parts of her counseling sessions.

The recurring vision of the partially naked man, which Lynette saw as a buried memory, was still a predominant worry for me. And one day, I had another memory of a conversation I had with my mother when I was about ten years old. It was an ominous warning. I wondered if these two things were linked. Not being an open family when it came to discussion of anything sexual, my mother's idea of the "mother and daughter facts-of-life talk" never got beyond menstruation. So it was particularly jarring when one day, out of nowhere, my mom blurted out, "Do you know what sex is?" Her inquiry left me slack-jawed. The only time sex was mentioned in my family was as part of a dirty joke. It's a good thing I was sitting down at the kitchen table, or I probably would have fallen "ass over tea kettle", as the saying goes.

"Yes," I said, my voice quivering. "I see the cows, even the turkeys doing it all the time," then I giggled nervously.

"John Meredith has been caught having sex with young girls," Mom replied. There was a long uneasy pause. "I want you to make sure you stay away from him," she said sternly. John Meredith was the neighbor from up the road past Grandpa and Grandma's place. He was Larry's dad, a boy who came over to play sometimes.

"Make sure you *never* take a ride from him if you're walking to Grandpa's!" Mom cautioned. This seemed like a strange request because I could never remember a time when he had offered me a ride. There was another long, uncomfortable pause. "He has been having sex with young girls so stay away from him, do you understand?" Mom pushed. The tone in her voice had left no doubt she meant business. "Don't *ever* go with him!" Mom was now yelling.

"I won't! I won't," I cried, and got up and ran out, slamming the screen door behind me.

I recalled a few other stories about him. He had been a horrible drinker often becoming abusive with his family. His wife ran a mile and a half in the middle of winter seeking help from my grandparents. It made perfect sense that he was a person I should fear.

Soon after I shared this information with Lynette, another significant memory revealed itself. I had this flashback on the way home from a counseling session. This was the recurring vision of the man with his hat on sideways, pants down around his ankles; only now I could see his erect penis. I glanced up and for an instant I saw his face. This was not the neighbor Mom warned me about. This was a handsome young man. He was smooth shaven, had hazel eyes and a thick head of dark hair showing out from the cap. I felt like I should know him. If I did know him perhaps I could find him in our old photo albums. I had taken quite an interest in gathering older pictures from both Dad's and Mom's sides of the family, so I had many on hand.

I got out the books and began thumbing through them. I had seen them all before, many times, over the last several months but today the sense of foreboding was thick. Of course I knew who this was. It was a much, much younger version, but the same man. Carefully, slowly, I flipped back through the pictures, through the years until I got to my Mom and Dad's wedding picture, the one with just the two of them. I stopped and stared at the young, handsome face in the picture: the smooth-shaven face and the head of dark, thick hair. It was the same dark, thick hair that jutted out from under the slightly askew cap.

I froze and so did everything else around me. I could hear myself breathing but everything else was muffled, like I was under a blanket. I had opened a door into a world from which there was no return. I could never have envisioned what would happen next. A line had been drawn in the sand and nothing, from this point forward, would ever be the same again.

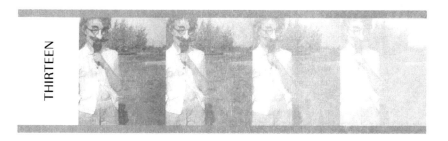

# THIRTEEN

# Drawn Together for a Divine Purpose

As difficult as it was, I kept all of this a secret. My outside world was pretty much as it was before I started seeing Lynette. I had to hold it all together and keep up my routine of wife and mother. Inside, however, my world was swirling like a hurricane, churning up events I could not have imagined possible. No one in my life—not even Rick—knew what was happening except my therapist. I was away working or doing so much volunteer work that he never questioned where I was.

It was so difficult keeping this locked up. I longed to have a friend I could confide in. *Maybe I could talk to Sylvia*, I thought. I had only known her a couple of years but we had hit it off right away. She was ten years or so younger than I was but she had a lot of tough life experiences that gave her perspective beyond her years. She was a single mom raising three young children on her own. She was from the same farming area as I was and so we knew a lot of the same people.

It was an easy and comfortable relationship, one with instant trust; she liked to talk but she was not a gossip. Sylvia was also new to the church—accepting Christ as an adult, as I had—and that gave us something else in common. We attended the same church women's group, the same Wednesday night Bible study, and her children were part of the kids' program that I led. When we were together we often joked about being kindred spirits drawn together by Divine purpose.

I called Sylvia and asked her to come over for a visit. Not only did I feel the need to confide in her but I also thought that, since her family was from the same district as mine, perhaps they might know some of my family history.

Sylvia came over that afternoon. I filled her in on what had been occurring in my life. My friend sat strangely quiet for quite some time as I told her about seeing a therapist, the night terrors, and the strange visions. I described the strange and consuming fear I had of the unknown, a fear like I had never experienced before. I continued talking and she just listened. I described how I had nearly no early childhood memories, that looking in a family photo album was liking looking at someone else's life. Then I told her about coming to the conclusion that I may have been abused by my own father.

Finally she spoke. "I don't know how to say this, but I know something about your dad. I feel God wants me to tell you what I know. First, we need to pray!"

"You know something about my d-dad?" I stuttered in utter disbelief.

"Please," Sylvia said, "let's pray."

Bowing my head, I sat in complete bewilderment. I nodded in agreement as Sylvia prayed: "Heavenly Father, we know you are a gracious and loving God and we ask for your loving direction for every word I speak and everything I am about to share today and Lord, I pray for Chris that you give her the strength she needs to deal with what she is about to learn and I ask that true healing comes from all of this. In Jesus' name I pray, amen."

She barely drew a breath before she said, "Chris, you weren't the only person your dad molested."

"What, what?" I said, mouth agape. Had I heard right? Was she confirming that my dad *had* molested me? And that he had hurt other people as well? Suddenly my head was pounding. I felt perplexed, angry, annoyed, excited all at once. And a crowd of voices seemed to be all talking at once: *"It can't be true." "Of course it is." "How does Sylvia know any of this?" "Who else? Who else?"*

Sylvia started in, "This is a story that I'd heard about for years. It is difficult to tell but you need to hear it." I bristled as she continued, "My mother had some relatives who lived just a short distance from town, between there and your family farm. They had twin boys, sweet, shy boys. One spring day, when the boys were about nine, they were walking home from town. Your dad was on his way home, driving a green John Deere tractor pulling an empty wagon. He'd probably hauled a load of grain to the local elevator and was on his return trip. Apparently, he'd spent some time in the beer parlor celebrating the birth of his first child—you. Your mom was still in the hospital with you."

She took a sip of water, cleared her throat and continued, "When he reached the boys he stopped. He said, 'I have something to show you. Come with me.' Then he got down from the tractor. 'Come see, and I will give you a ride the rest of the way home.' He took one of the boy's hands and led him a way into the trees, the brother followed. He stopped and undid his zipper and exposed himself to the two frightened kids. 'Just touch it and I will give you a treat.'

"They both turned and ran. Your dad caught one of them. 'Never mind,' he consoled them. 'I will give you a ride home. Don't be scared.' He sat them on a narrow ledge on the front of the grain wagon. He didn't go very far when he hit a bump and one of the brothers fell off. The wagon tire ran over the boy's head killing him instantly. My mother always felt that your dad had put the boys' lives in jeopardy—on purpose—so no one would find out."

Pausing, Sylvia then said softy, "That's all I know."

Sylvia and I sat quietly for a while, letting everything sink in. "I am so sorry," Sylvia said. "I wasn't sure if I should tell you or not."

"Don't be sorry," I told her, "I needed to know and I am glad I found out from you."

"If you want to know more, you can get a hold of my mom," she offered. "She can answer your questions. I think she even has some newspaper clippings." Sylvia hugged me and then left me sitting at my kitchen table in a state of complete shock.

Once more I sat shaking and crying while looking out my kitchen window. My beautiful garden and flowers, the scenic countryside, didn't lend me any comfort.

My time with Sylvia that day would prove to be a pivotal point in the recovery of more memories and in the filling in of crucial points in the memories I had. More importantly it confirmed what all the voices inside my head most assuredly knew: my father had, indeed, sexually molested me.

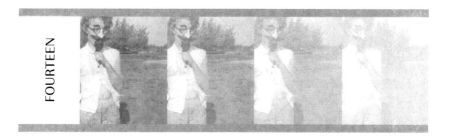

FOURTEEN

# *Grace and Forgiveness*

My mind flooded with questions. Had my father really tried to abuse the twin boys? Had he been responsible for one of them dying? Was that all to the story? What other secrets? Who else knew? I felt like I was walking through someone else's nightmare—only it wasn't someone else's. It was mine and, damn it, I was going to find out what everyone else knew!

I made a call to Sylvia's parents and made arrangements to see them the next morning. I was nervous as I drove the ten miles to their farm but I had a strange new resolve to dig in and do what it took to get to the bottom of this. In some ways I felt like an investigative reporter. I was gathering facts—facts that confirmed what Sylvia had told me.

They were very kind to me, telling me what they knew and felt. They had little to add to what Sylvia had said only that there had been a court case and as far as they knew Dad had walked away with no repercussions. They said facts about that were not clear. They had heard speculation of my grandfather selling some property to bail his son out of trouble. There may have been some truth to that as other sources told me of the sale of a Caterpillar tractor at that same time. As far as anything from the newspapers, all they had was the obituary of the young boy who had been killed.

"There were some other rumors, too, but I only heard about them, didn't know anyone involved," said Sylvia's mother. "We heard he molested a young girl just south of here."

Another story emerged later about my dad's involvement in a hit-and-run accident that killed someone. Sylvia's parents, along with relatives and an old friend of her dad's, had confirmed this. Apparently this had happened before Dad and Mom had gotten married. In all these cases when I looked to find out why he was never held accountable, the answer would always come back: his parents would do whatever it took to bail him out of trouble, never letting him be accountable for actions.

Having finished my visit with Sylvia's parents, I sat in my car in their driveway. My composure and confidence were gone. I began perspiring; there was a pain in my stomach, coming in waves. I was so very, very tired. I needed to get home.

Suddenly, I was in my house but I could not remember getting there. I needed to sleep. The boys wouldn't be home from school for another couple hours so I crawled into bed and drifted off right away, awaking only to the sound of the school bus in the yard and the kids coming home.

The next day the visit with Sylvia's parents floated in my mind like a dream, far off and hazy. I knew the mother of those twin boys. She was a sweet older lady. I used to see her around town but hadn't now for quite some time. I wondered, *Did that lady look at me and know. Who knew?* Sylvia's parents told me that she had moved to a community thirty miles away to be near two of her daughters.

I decided I needed to visit her. Why exactly, I wasn't sure; maybe to make a connection with this lady on whom my father had visited so much pain. I found her number in the phone book and sat looking at it. An hour passed before I actually dialed it.

The phone rang four times before a small, frail voice answered, "Hello." It was real. She existed. I wanted to scream, to run, to hide, to make it all disappear and I wanted to know more; so many confusing thoughts and feelings but still I knew I had to proceed.

"Yes, hello," she said again.

"Hello," I said, "Is this Mrs. Peters?"

"Yes," she again replied in a soft, shaky voice.

"My name is Christine Ducommun, do you remember the name?"

"Who did you say you were?" she inquired. The quiet hung in the air for what seemed an eternity.

I replied, "I think you know something about my family. I don't want to upset anyone. I just am trying to fill in some details in my own life. Would that be okay?"

The frail voice responded, "Why don't you come tomorrow afternoon, right after lunch. My daughters will be here."

"That's fine," I replied and we agreed on 1:30 PM.

I was so anxious about meeting this lady. I certainly didn't want to cause her family any more pain but I just had to meet her. I had to put the pieces together. The little town she had moved to was thirty miles away. The drive seemed endless. The dotted white lines seemed to stretch out far beyond their normal reach. I had taken a couple of extra tranquillizers as an added precaution but stopped at a convenience store on the way and bought five chocolate bars, a package of processed luncheon meat and a carton of chocolate milk, all of which I gobbled down in just a matter of a few miles. Food had always been a source of pleasure, and since I had started digging around in my past and unearthing memories, it became a means of comfort too. "Oh, well," I heard a voice say out loud. "I gained two pounds last week, and four this week so far—what's a few more hundred calories?"

I pulled into the lady's driveway. I felt as if I was out of my body, watching myself walk up to the tiny white house, like I was directing a movie in slow motion. I knocked at the door where the woman's two daughters met me. At first the welcome was cool and guarded. I got the feeling that they didn't completely trust me, but they seemed curious enough to put up with me. They must be wondering what I wanted. They certainly made it very clear that they were very protective of their mother, if not in what they said than certainly in their body language.

I proceeded to explain to them about what I believed was my own sexual abuse, and that I was just beginning to try to understand how it had impacted me. I wanted to learn how to heal from it. I told of how my friend Sylvia had shared with me what she knew about my dad and that was what had brought me to their mother's doorstep. I talked without interruption and felt like I was babbling—and at double the speed of normal conversation. The two daughters kept getting up from the kitchen table and fussing around: more tea, mores cookies, more napkins. I could tell this was hard on them. Their mother, on the other hand, sat very still. She was hanging on every word. Occasionally her pale blue eyes misted over and she blinked away the moisture.

"I am so sorry for the loss of your son," I said. I looked at her, now fragile and elderly in her eighties. Though it had happened so long ago, I knew from my own experience that you never get over the loss of a child—and the manner in which she lost her son was simply hideous. "I don't want to cause you any more pain. I am so sorry for what my dad did." My comforting words changed the atmosphere. The daughters' expressions softened and they dropped their arms, which had been crossed defensively.

"You have nothing to apologize for," Mrs. Peters said and both daughters agreed. They all expressed such compassion and care. "After all you were just a baby," she continued. Inwardly I breathed a sigh of relief.

Many times that afternoon they told me how I must never blame myself and never again apologize for Dad, saying it was not my fault. I was humbled by Mrs. Peters' grace and compassion.

Then she retold in her own words the heart-wrenching story that Sylvia had shared with me. She was so tiny and fragile, with thin wisps of white hair surrounding her face, transparent and pink with age. The story was not much different than what she has already heard, the facts varying little, but so profound coming from her lips. She spared little. She still didn't cry, but her eyes misted over occasionally and she'd take the odd pause to compose herself. Her daughters cried openly, often standing and walking away.

She stopped and looked directly at me, "I know how old you are," she said. "Do you know how I know?"

"No, how?" I asked, trembling.

"You were a newborn when this happened, still in the hospital. I have thought about you many times over the years, when the anniversary of my son's death comes around." I was flabbergasted. For nearly four decades, a woman I didn't even know existed had thought of me every year. How strange it must be for her to meet with me face to face like this and relive this horrible event.

"Did anyone in my family ever make any effort to apologize? Did anyone ever say they were sorry?" I asked.

"No one," Mrs. Peters replied, "No one ever even talked to me, but he paid for the funeral—that was because the judge made him."

"Really?" I gasped, momentarily at a loss for words, "Can you tell me about that?" I wanted to cry, to be sick, I was shaking; then, an unexpected calm enveloped me like a warm quilt.

"I don't remember much, and my brother-in-law looked after most of that for me. My husband was away sick again," she says. Then Mrs. Peters recounted a sad story of mental illness in her own family and an abusive husband who went insane and had to be locked away because of his violent episodes.

She told how her surviving twin son confided in her about the attempted sexual abuse at the hands of Dad. "I brought him before the judge and he told what happened." This was 1952. These were not days of open communication, where children freely discussed sex with their parents, much less felt safe enough to share something like this.

"Do you think my dad wanted to hurt your son?" I asked, not sure where such a stupid question would come from.

"I never blamed him, never thought he wanted to kill him, but that other stuff," she said and she stopped and shook her head, eyes misting over again, "Why would a man want to do that? I never will understand that."

Her daughters were crying openly again and I realized they would have been young girls when this happened. How drastically their lives were affected by this tragedy; I wondered if they ever talked about it over the years.

I was there the entire afternoon. I sensed it was time to go, but walking out the door was a very hard thing. My shoes felt like they had lead weights in them, and again I was exhausted.

Later that spring, about two weeks after my fortieth birthday, I was in town picking up the mail. I sat in my car in front of the post office, sorting through the flyers and the bills as I typically did. There was a card. I thought, obviously someone was late remembering my birthday. Those were always fun to get. "Hmm. I wonder who sent this to me?" I wondered out loud. It was a very pretty card with a simple greeting, wishing me a happy birthday, signed by Mrs. Peters and her two daughters. "It was so good to meet you," they wrote. "We wish you much peace and healing."

I was so touched by this gesture. Tears rolled down my cheeks as I thought of the strange bond I had shared with these ladies. They were the very definition of grace and forgiveness.

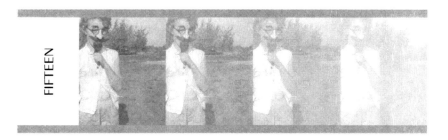

# FIFTEEN

# Reconstructing the Past

That summer, while my sons filled their days with Bible camp, swimming lessons and friends, and my husband kept busy working many overtime hours for a local farmer, I spent every spare minute trying to reconstruct—or for that matter *construct*—my past. It became vitally important to find out what my family appeared like from the outside; anything I could get my hands on, something, anything, to build on, to give this family some substance. Fortunately my friend Sylvia often looked after my children while I was trying to put the pieces together.

My dad's first cousin Cathy and her husband, Bob, still lived in the same district. We had actually gotten to know each other quite well, having served on a couple of different community causes. They were next in line for a visit. Question by question, more pieces of the puzzle began to fall into place.

Once again I began by explaining that I had been sexually abused by my father but that I had so few memories of my childhood that I was hoping to put some pieces together. They were a little hesitant at first but little by little stories began to unfold. They, too, knew of the boy being killed and of Grandpa selling things at the same time to keep his son out of jail.

The more they talked, the clearer the picture of my father's family became—a family of deep dysfunction. "He drank a lot from the time he was very young," said Cathy. "He was constantly getting into trouble but he never had to take responsibility for his actions."

I told Cathy that my mother had warned me about Mr. Meredith, the neighbor to our north, and that how initially I thought he had been my abuser. Their response to that was very interesting. "Mr. Meredith was no saint, that's for sure," said Bob. "He was an alcoholic and beat his wife. He was already tainted and that allowed your father to take advantage by deflecting any suspicion about wrongdoing Meredith's way. Mr. Meredith was an obvious and believable target."

"Some time ago, when you were very young, Mr. Meredith was accused of trying to rape a neighbor girl. She was about ten years older than you. Your dad claimed to have saved her and he was made out to be a hero. After that, the Meredith's left town and we never saw or heard from them again."

"That was what my mother warned me about," I said. She said Mr. Meredith tried to rape the neighbor girl.

I watched their faces as they looked across the table at me. I could visibly see the sickening truth take hold as the horrible realization sunk in. Having lived only a few miles down the road, they had known me from the time I had been a red-headed, freckle-faced little girl. They knew my dad and my mom. They knew my grandparents.

"We knew he was a sick person," Cathy said.

"We knew he had been in a lot of trouble when he was young. We knew he was a liar. We knew he had a drinking problem. We knew he worked you girls way too hard and we didn't like that," said Bob, shaken. They were crying now and hugging me.

"We didn't know . . . we didn't know he was doing *that!*" they said, their faces buried into their hands.

Incrementally, pieces of the flashbacks begin to form a picture and a couple memories began to take shape. They started out with little millisecond flashes—of scenes, sounds, smells, physical pain—and would build from there, with pieces added until either a partial or complete memory was formed.

"Your initial wounding happened when you were a child," Lynette explained to me one day. We need to work on healing that inner child and I suspect this might clear up your early childhood memory problems.

We began by doing some visualization exercises where I would try to walk back in my memory until I was younger and younger. I also began a workbook entitled *The Wounded Heart: Hope for Adult Victims of Childhood Sexual Abuse* by Dr. Dan B. Allender, a Christian book which dealt specifically with the spiritual damage of victims of childhood sexual abuse. I felt driven to uncover what had happened and what was happening to me now. It seemed to make sense that going back and nurturing my inner child would help me in the present.

One of the first memories to come together with quite a bit of detail, even though fragmented, involved another victim. The timing of this memory was crucial because it helped me believe and accept that all this was rooted in reality, and that I wasn't crazy. It was the glue to my sanity. I was not making this up. This was not the figment of some warped, attention-starved lunatic. It also kept me from staying in a semi-permanent state of denial, however necessary that was as a means for occasional respite. The process was emotionally grueling and I often needed distance to comprehend it all.

This particular memory involved a boy named Larry, who was only a couple months older than me. I remembered he often came to play, especially that one summer. I was going into grade one and Mom and Dad had bought me my first two-wheel bike. I was so proud. I wasn't sure if it was brand new or not, but it was shiny silver and blue. They took it out of the truck when they got home and Dad pushed me a couple of times to get me started and then he went in the house. Many times my parents told the story of how

I came into the house that afternoon, with bruised and scraped knees and elbows, proudly relating how I had mastered the skill of riding the two-wheeler.

Larry came to visit on a very oversized tricycle, and I felt very proud and maybe a little glib that I now rode a two-wheeler. Along with that ridiculously oversized tricycle, I remember Larry being a skinny boy with dirty blond hair and a runny nose. He was never very happy and was always whining or crying about something or another.

The last play date I had with Larry was on a hot summer day. We are playing behind a row of red square grain bins. I remember playing there a lot when it got hot. It was cooler there, in the shade and in the tall, lush green grass that tickled my legs. I am wearing shorts and so is Larry, which emphasizes his really skinny legs and boney knees.

I am not sure where Mom is. She works very hard and has a big garden to tend to, along with milking cows, raising the chickens, ducks and geese, and even driving the tractor. I have one little sister, who is about three years old. Maybe Mom is with her. Our black-and-white dog, Sport, is with us. His tail is wagging and he is panting, which makes it look like he is smiling.

Suddenly he is just there, standing between two of the red grain bins, watching. I see him first and freeze. Larry is caught completely off guard. He turns to see what has happened to me and why I am not talking to him. My dad reaches out and grabs him by the scruff of the neck. Larry is taken so completely by surprise that he flails in midair. I am backed up tight against one of the grain bins. My knees are tucked up under my chin and I am hiding my head in my arms. Larry lets out a yelp and Dad quickly slaps a hand over his mouth, snarling something under his breath about being quiet if he knows what's good for him. He pushes Larry into the long lush green grass, grabbing his shorts and yanking them off.

I peek out, past Larry to Sport, who has his head cocked to one side in bewilderment. I put my head back into my arms. Larry cries out again and I know that's a bad thing. He

76          Living with Multiple Personalities

needs to be quiet. I peek again and see a stick. I think it's a stick. I see Dad pull Larry's little pink thing and grab his bum. Dad has his pants down.

Suddenly I hear someone singing, I concentrate on the singing. Then it stops. Now I feel dark and angry, and a voice is saying, "Run, run!" Just as quickly as the anger came on it's over, and suddenly it's quiet again. Now I feel warm and safe.

Is that a stick? It looks like a hammer, but it's not a hammer. Larry has his face in the grass. He is not making any sounds now. There are tears running into the grass. He is shaking. His whole body is shaking.

Looking up, I see Dad standing directly in front of me now. His pants are around his ankles. "It's always better to be a good girl. Always better!" says a comforting, grandmotherly voice. Who said that? I wonder. It didn't sound like Dad.

I look past again and see Sport, still looking so curious. His head still cocked. Maybe he will bark and maybe someone will hear him. He doesn't. Dad waves and gestures at me; I can't move. I see Larry in the grass.

Someone says, "You must go."

Then another person shouts, "NO! Be good. Good girls must listen."

Daddy grabs the front of my blouse, and just as he does I hear someone calling him terrible names. This makes me really frightened, and I want him to stop, because it can only get me into terrible trouble and I will be hit again.

"No, I won't go!" an angry voice yells. Dad slaps me, hard across the head.

I need to be quiet. It's essential for survival. He shoves my face into his crotch and barks instructions. I have heard them before. I obey. Daddy reaches for me, and pulls off my little pink flowered panties, then pokes and probes with dirty and angry fingers.

There is an old woman holding me, stroking my hair, soothing me with her beautiful velvet voice, "Oh my darling, oh my darling, oh my darling Clementine..."

Dad moans and rocks back and forth. I know it will soon be over. "I will hold you, and comfort you and sing to you," says the grandmotherly voice inside my head. "Listen, honey, listen to the song you love: "Oh my darling, oh my darling, oh my darling, Clementine . . . you were lost and then I found you. . . ."

Then the excruciating pain is over. He leaves me in the mess he has created. "Don't ever tell anyone about this or I'll kill you!" he sputters. I believe him. Larry goes home. Larry doesn't come to play again.

Working through this memory with Lynette took weeks. I would divulge only a few details at a time even though I knew more. The revelation of my childhood reality was a double-edged sword: I knew I was not going insane but the horrible truth of the abuse and speaking of it out loud was at times overwhelming. I feared that if I actually talked about these things that had happened the pain would be too big and would destroy me. Rationally I knew that wasn't the case, but reality was distorted for me. Sometimes insanity seemed preferable.

After some time had passed, Lynette and I decided to schedule a two-hour appointment to deal with the memory with Larry. I really wasn't looking forward to revisiting the incident. I looked around for the box of tissues, but knew I needed something to hold onto—something soft and comforting. Lynette frequently worked with children so there was an assortment of stuffed toys in a wicker basket in the corner. I settled on a soft pillow. Much of the long session was filled with gut-wrenching, childlike crying. I clutched the pillow, burying my face into it. "Should I take this home and wash it?" I asked Lynette, "Or should I just burn all the ugly memories I've spilled into it?"

I was completely shaken by the unearthing of this memory with Larry. Knowing that my father had so terribly abused me as a little girl was bad enough, but realizing he had also abused my friends added exponentially to my pain and the horror of what he had done. Yet I was hopeful that the time in counseling would heal the little girl within me, or at the very least help me purge the ghosts. It didn't, yet what it did do was a miracle in itself. It set up an even deeper trust with Lynette. I can't believe that my first impression of her was that I didn't think she looked like a therapist. I don't know what a therapist is supposed to look like but this tiny, young woman wasn't what I had envisioned. However, I couldn't have been more pleased with her. She had a quiet, comforting demeanor and spoke in a soft, soothing voice. Until that two hour session that little girl in me, the one I hadn't even known until this point in my life, had never before extended her hand to anyone outside; it truly was the beginning of the healing. I hadn't even begun to realize or understand the significance and the enormity of this step.

As Lynette would disclose to me later, however, some unusual behavior began to surface during this time of which I had no recollection. Apparently during some of my sessions I would speak as different little girls. They were distinct but all quite young and they would rapidly switch from one to another and back again. One little girl would cry and hide her head. Another would suddenly get up and dance around the room. Then there was another who would sulk in silence. It was very curious. Perhaps I had more than one inner child.

The memory with Larry also sparked a curiosity. I wondered what had become of him and felt a growing, almost desperate urge to try and find and connect with him. His family had moved away the fall after the incident behind the granaries. I was sure Larry had not even started school. His mom and older sister, who was at least ten years his senior, had remained in contact with my mom. They still had extended family in the area so I thought it might not be that hard to get in touch with them. At this point I had not shared any of what was going on with my mom or sisters so I tried to be as discreet as possible. It was all I could do to try to believe it myself. I certainly wasn't ready to explain it to them.

I had heard some rumors about Larry in the early 1980s, something about him joining the Ramakrishna movement in Toronto and then moving to Vancouver where he was apparently driving a taxi. I found out his sister had married a farmer in the southern part of the province. I got her address and very carefully put together a letter.

I worded the correspondence very carefully, explaining I had suffered sexual abuse at the hands of my father and had a memory that included my dad sexually abusing Larry as well. I said I was hoping to piece some other things together and perhaps make some contact with Larry. I added that I wished not to cause any heartache or distress. I fearfully mailed this letter and waited.

It took many weeks before I got a reply. Larry's older sister's letter was filled with compassion and sincere sympathy. She apologized for the length of time it had taken her to reply and admitted that it was because she had been in a state of shock. She also talked about how painful it had been for her to go back in her memories because of her own father's severe alcoholism and the emotional and verbal abuse her family suffered as a result of that. She did say that she had never suffered anything inappropriate at the hands of my father. However, she remembered a time when Larry was around five or six and had horrible nightmares. He would wake up screaming. They never did get to the bottom of what was wrong and eventually the nightmares stopped. She said that she and Larry were never very close. "Larry seems to be such as lost soul," she wrote, "and sadly I have lost all contact. My mother had received a postcard from him, saying he was moving to Alberta and then the next one she got from him was postmarked Ireland. That was seven years ago and no one has seen or heard from him since."

I felt utterly sad for this man. I wondered how my dad had altered the course of his life. Larry was important for another reason; he had played a role in another memory that included a different victim. I believe this incident happened the same summer as the one with just Larry and me. It would have been so good to talk to Larry, to help fill in the gaps.

This incident occurred in a building that Mom and Dad lived in temporarily when they were first married. When this episode took place it was being used as a granary. It had some partial cupboards in one corner.

I am cowering in one corner. Larry is there too. An older girl is there. She must be older because she is much bigger than Larry and me.

She is lying on her back on the cupboard. Dad is standing at the end of the cupboard between her legs. He is rocking back and forth and moaning. The same moaning I have heard so many times. It's like no one knows I am there and I am happy for that.

There are many voices cackling away in my head, but at least it's only me who can hear them. It's always good to be quiet. Then, suddenly, they all start chattering, making a lot of noise. I wish they would stop, because I'm going to get hit by my dad if they continue this.

Now there is more noise; this time coming from outside my head. The door to the granary has opened and someone else is there. There is another man in the room. There is screaming, yelling. It's the girl on the cupboard. She is grabbing for Dad and he is pushing me out the granary door.

I realize that the other man is Larry's dad. That doesn't make any sense! Why would Larry's dad be there? My dad whispers in my ear, "Tell and you die!"

I hear familiar voices in my head. They hush and protect. One is singing to me. Then it is quiet. I am in the sunshine. It hurts my eyes.

"Get in the house," Dad growls and pushes me in through the porch door.

I am inside now. I hear the sound of a truck starting up and I watch through the living room window. It is Larry's dad's truck and he drives away. Larry's dirty blond head is barely visible in the rear window. The truck turns north, toward Larry's house.

I hear the sound of another vehicle start up. I peek above the windowsill again. My dad drives out of the yard and turns the other direction. The older girl is in his truck. It looks like Arlene, Dad's cousin. But how, why?

We had other neighbors to the south, less than half a mile away, the opposite direction of Larry's home. They were Dad's aunt and uncle and they had two girls who were Dad's first cousins. Arlene was one and I remember her causing all kinds of problems, eventually becoming so uncontrollable she had been institutionalized. I believe she was only sixteen at the time. My parents spoke of her in later years, Dad saying fondly, "They should have left her alone. There was nothing wrong with her other than being a little oversexed."

I had a very clear recollection of a time when this cousin had stayed at our house. There had been some kind of family event, possibly a birthday or maybe even Christmas. Arlene was typically released home for a few days for special occasions but she had refused to stay with her parents and wanted to stay at my home. I recalled my parents saying how she had a crush on Dad. In the course of this short one- or two-day visit with us, she made it clear she wanted to get rid of my mom and us children so she could have Dad to herself. Finally it became apparent that this was a dangerous situation and, after consultation between my parents, grandparents and Arlene's parents, they summoned a doctor from a neighboring community to help get her under control and take her back to the Provincial Mental Institution.

I recall the night spent waiting for the doctor. My father stationed himself across the doorway to our bedrooms while the family tried to sleep, but twice Arlene made it past him, and Mom and Dad would have to bodily force her back downstairs. The doctor arrived the next morning and again I recalled a huge fuss and bits and pieces of conversations. There was discussion of how smart she had been about the medications, knowing exactly what the doctor was going to give her and convincing him that she needed more.

I suspected this girl to be the one in the granary. Most of her adult life was spent in the Provincial Mental Institution and during that time she had several trial visits home but inevitably she would lose control and there would be some kind of fiasco, from her threatening her mom with a butcher knife to running down Main Street in her pajamas.

After many years of institutional living she did become well enough to be placed in a community day-work program. In fact, she met and fell in love with a rather nice fellow. Many wonderful reports came home of how happy she was and of how well this man was treating her, and it seemed perhaps she had found a small slice of peace at last. While she was married to this gentleman she actually felt strong enough to visit the old hometown, but once again the old demons from the past would give her no rest and those visits disintegrated into disasters. Those were her last visits and she never returned again. Arlene and her husband did have several happy years together but that slipped away as did her mental stability and once again she returned to the institution.

I longed to talk to her. Was she, indeed, one of Dad's victims? I couldn't bring myself to actually face her without contacting her immediate family first, so I decided to send a letter to the closest remaining family member, her sister Sherry, who was only two years older than Arlene. Sherry had moved to British Columbia, two provinces away. Once again I carefully worded my letter, explaining my sexual abuse and asking if there was any possibility that this had happened to Arlene as well.

Months passed and I had resigned myself to never hearing back from Sherry when one Sunday morning the phone rang. "Hello Chris, this is Sherry, Arlene's sister. I received your letter and I am sorry that I did not reply to you sooner." She sounded nervous. Strangely, this was the same response as I had gotten from Larry's sister. I went on to explain that I had been so young when all this had occurred and that of course little was discussed with me. She went on to say though that sexual abuse had definitely been a part of her sister's problem. This was never discussed openly in those days, of course, but she had overheard her parents talking.

Her assumption had always been that it had been the neighbor to the north, because of his terrible drinking reputation. She had not once considered that my father, her own cousin, had done anything inappropriate to her.

"Do you think it would be possible for me to visit Arlene? I'd just like to ask her a few questions and I promise I won't upset her." I said.

Sherry answered, "I really don't think that is a good idea. I can understand why you would want to, but what's the point, really? My sister is so far removed from reality that you wouldn't get anything out of the visit but frustration."

I took a deep breath, trying to conceal my disappointment. "Okay. I respect your decision," I said. "Thank you again for calling me."

I made one more visit to Cathy and Bob, the relatives who still lived in the community. I wanted to know if they remembered or knew anything of this cousin or of this story. They knew the story, but it had a different twist. The evil rapist was not my father but rather Larry's dad, the horrible, abusive alcoholic to the north. My dad had saved the young girl cousin. What a clever manipulation of events. What a sitting duck our neighbor to the north had been. The only real witnesses: two terrified kids who were not going to say anything for fear of death, and a young girl desperately in love with her attacker. Once again a look of utter disgust came over them as the reality of how they had been duped by this sick, perverted man came to light.

This was a time of great turmoil for me; a time when so many horrible realizations were happening and yet I couldn't bring myself to include my family. I really couldn't imagine letting my mom and sisters know, and neither could I involve my husband. I was afraid of not being believed, and my husband and my dad had been close. Of course my sons were too young to deal with this. I suppose I needed to be sure before telling anyone. I curiously sought out more information that proved my dad was an abuser and the longer I kept this secret the more I felt like a traitor. After all what good could come of this knowledge? My family of origin never admitted that anything might be amiss; even something as normal as dealing with a crop failure was covered up. It was an unwritten rule that what was family business stayed just that. We were, for all intents and purposes, the quintessential honest, hardworking family and that was all the information that was necessary. I was a product of my environment and I felt guilty sneaking around and searching for the truth. The idea of revealing my findings also caused the same feeling. Secrecy was absolutely paramount.

My now-weekly therapy sessions with Lynette were my lifeline and I looked forward to them. There were days that were more difficult than others, but when I felt like I was going to drop off the side of a cliff, scrambling to get a toehold on reality, Lynette was reaching over the top and offering me her hand. By now there was not a shred of doubt left in my mind that my father had been my abuser, and that I had been one of who knows how many victims of his perversion. Uncovering the details was one thing; the healing that needed to take place was quite another—and I realized I needed to get on with that part now that the big mystery had been solved. I needed to put all this behind me and go forward. I wanted desperately to be rid of the flashbacks, the night terrors and have some peace of mind.

"Lynette, I just want to move on. I want to feel normal, whatever that is. I'm desperate to be rid of all of this," I told her.

Lynette nodded her head. Somehow just a look from her could put me at ease. "This is a long, painful process, Chris. Revealing all of these memories is traumatic, which is why your mind buried them. For our next session, I want to give you something different for homework. Try to recall something good from your childhood and be ready to discuss it the next time we get together."

After all this turmoil and pain, I silently wondered, *Was there anything good about my childhood? Will I ever be free from this secret?*

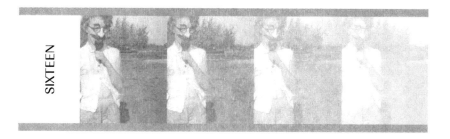

# SIXTEEN

# Lilacs and Enduring Love

After so many dark memories, it was nice to have something good to bring to therapy, and I thanked Lynette for knowing that I needed a break from all the horror. I brought a memory of my great-grandmother Annie. I would revive it often in the years to come when things would get particularly painful.

I was fourteen when Great-Grandma Annie passed away, so my memories of her were very vivid. She was my dad's grandmother on his mother's side of the family. She was born in England and every bit a proper lady. After she was too old to live by herself, she moved in with my grandparents, who lived just down the road less than a half mile. My grandmother grumbled a lot about this arrangement but, mind you, Grandmother spent most of her time grumbling about something.

Great-Grandma Annie was deaf. If you spoke clearly, slowly and directly to her, she was very good at reading lips so you could communicate. She also carried a pad so you could write to her. She always wore pretty dresses, usually with a white sweater over top. She always had on white stockings and very sturdy, sensible shoes. I loved her hugs. Her skin was so soft and she smelled good—like soap.

I didn't have many early childhood memories but there was one that included her. It was a warm summer day; I was eight years old and my mom had given me permission to go to my grandparents. I knew Great-Grandma Annie was there, so I was very excited. I loved visiting with her and hearing her stories about life in England. Skipping down the road, I hoped we would have a picnic under the huge lilac tree in the front yard. That was always so much fun. One of my favorite things to do was kicking off my shoes and going barefoot in the creeping Charlie. My mom called creeping Charlie an awful weed. I had a completely different opinion. It grew thick and short to the ground and had gorgeous little purple flowers. It felt so neat between my toes. Sometimes I would lay flat on my stomach so I could see the flowers right up close.

When I got to my grandparents' house I burst through the door, my face bright and shining with anticipation.

"Hi, Great-Grandma!" I shouted. Great-Grandma Annie's face lit up with a big smile when she saw me.

"Good morning Chrissy!" she beamed. "Come here, my beloved child." I ran to her and gave her a big hug, falling into her soft folds.

Grandma was grumping around in the background, complaining about something or another. Great-Grandma never paid much attention to her, either because she couldn't hear her—or maybe because she was impervious to all that negativity.

Leaning back, and holding Great-Grandma's hands, I mouthed my words carefully, "Can we have a picnic?"

"We *will* have a picnic," Great-Grandma answered. "You run along and wait outside. I will be there shortly," she said.

Out under the big lilac tree I ran in circles, waving my arms and weaving around like a bird. Then I dropped to the ground, deeply enthralled with the petite purple flowers of the creeping Charlie underworld. There were bugs of every description. I loved them all. A daddy long-legs scurried ahead of my quick little fingers. Then there was the prize catch: it was magnificent, a yellow and black striped, fuzzy longhaired caterpillar. I lifted my head and saw Great-Grandma coming from the house.

I ever so carefully picked up the caterpillar so as not to hurt him. His fuzzy hair tickled my hand as he marched up my arm. "Look," I said and proudly displayed my new friend.

"Isn't he a grand one!" Great-Grandma proclaimed. "May I see him closer?" I slowly and ever so carefully brought him about so Great-Grandma could have a closer look. The caterpillar wriggled and I giggled as he continued his march up my arm.

"I think it's time we let him go," Granny said, "time for our picnic, and time to wash our hands."

I walked into the yard and carefully let my little friend go. I turned and ran into the house to get ready for the picnic. I hoped Grandma wouldn't grouch at me; luckily I didn't see her. Back in the yard Great-Grandma had everything ready. On the picnic table was an elegant white crocheted tablecloth. I recalled that someone once said it was a pineapple pattern. I didn't know what that meant exactly, but it sure looked fancy. I knew Granny liked it. She brought out a glass pitcher, painted with bright red and yellow tulips, filled with lemonade. The drinking glasses had the same flowered pattern on them. There were also little glass plates for the cookies. Great-Grandma always poured the lemonade and served the cookies; we had a picnic like proper English ladies.

After we were done eating Granny went back into the house and brought out her Scrabble game. She had been teaching me how to play. I loved Scrabble and her crossword puzzles. Sometimes I would sit and watch her do the puzzles and listen while Granny interspersed her puzzle-solving with her stories of being a little girl. Today was Scrabble day. I felt like a princess.

This memory proved to be one I clung to in the years to come, a brief but wonderful respite from the many other memories I had to sort through and deal with. Sometimes when things got darkest, when I was most afraid, I would sit and imagine the smell of lilac flowers or the feel of soft lawn under my feet, and I would be transported to a time with Great-Grandma Annie. I could feel my whole being relax, and warmth spread over me. Other times the mere appearance of lilac trees or fancy crocheted doilies would send a comforting wonderful peace through me and conjure up the fragrance of freshly washed hands and a feeling of enduring love.

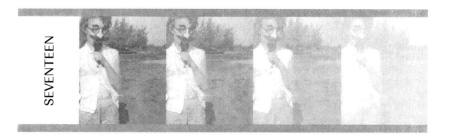

# SEVENTEEN

# From One into Many

Lynette's therapeutic focus continued down the path of resurrecting childhood memories. However, as time wore on the strange occurrence of me behaving as different children, which started in our session to analyze the "Larry memory," continually cropped up in our new sessions. We'd be in the middle of a visualization exercise when, suddenly, I'd break out into fits of giggling. At other times I'd pout, refusing to speak. On other occasions I'd get up and dance around the room. I often wouldn't remember any of this.

Then there were the other bizarre episodes at home. "Something strange happened to me this week," I told her one day. "I found a childhood picture of myself, tacked to my bulletin board by the phone. Next to it, written in a young child's scrawl, was a message 'Take me home,'" I said nervously. It was like I had traded one set of weird occurrences—the flashbacks, the night terrors— for another. I felt like I was living in some strange mystery movie.

"Who do you think put it there?" she asked.

"I haven't any idea," I answered. My family does not know about you or our sessions. I just recently gathered together these photos. Even if it were my sons who put up the picture—which is just about impossible—their handwriting is not like this. The note was written by a very young child, someone who is just beginning to learn how to write."

Lynette scribbled something on her notepad but I somehow sensed that she was troubled. "Our time is up for today," she said. "Just keep working through the book this week, as you have been, and we'll begin to sort this out at our next session."

The following week, Lynette looked at me earnestly and said, "Chris, we have been meeting for some time now and have made amazing progress in unlocking things from your past and finding out why you were having nightmares and recurring visions. It's been a tough, difficult road with much work yet to be done." I nodded in agreement. "But something more is happening here. Something for which I don't feel adequately trained. The instances where you speak as a little girl—actually several little girls—are happening more and more. I don't believe this is merely an inner child issue. It's as though you are more than one person."

I stared at her with my mouth agape while she continued. "I've done a lot of reading and research and I suspect that what you might have is known as dissociative identity disorder, or DID."

"Dissociative . . . *what?*" I said. I had no idea what she was talking about but it sounded serious.

"Dissociative identity disorder. It used to be called multiple personality disorder," she explained, "when the mind splits off into several personalities, or alters, due to repeated traumatic episodes, in order to protect itself."

I just stared at the wall, absolutely speechless. I could hardly process what she was telling me; my head was spinning. "Anyway, Chris," she continued, "I think that you have come as far with me as you can. I really feel that you need to find a therapist with more experience, someone with more knowledge of this disorder, who can better help you."

"No," I flatly refused. "Lynette, you have been my savior. I just don't trust anyone else. I can't imagine starting over with someone new—especially not now!"

She tried her best to make her case for someone better trained but I stood firm. She said, "Okay, what if we involve another therapist to assist me, perhaps in a consulting capacity?" It sounded fair and reasonable so I said yes. "But first I'd like to set up an appointment with you to see a psychiatrist who can confirm or disprove my diagnosis."

I agreed to that. Shortly thereafter I went to Dr. Matthews for an analysis. I saw him only once and the report he sent back was that he agreed with Lynette on the DID diagnosis. While at first I was shocked, when I began to think back it all seemed to make sense. For years I had heard voices in my head. I had just assumed that everybody had this. After all, we all think to ourselves to some extent. I just assumed that I had a more active brand of this than other people since no one had ever told me otherwise. What seemed new and different, especially since the unearthing of the Larry memory, was the number of voices all speaking at the same time and my lapses in memory in the present time.

With an established diagnosis in hand, Lynette consulted with a psychologist in the same community who was a specialist in the diagnosis of mental health issues. His role was to assist Lynette in some of the more complicated sessions where the little girls presented.

Many sessions were spent allowing the children to express themselves, with Lynette interacting with them, playing, laughing, and holding them, whatever it took. Trust deepened between Lynette and me, and the child alters. Slowly but surely each of them, who were almost one dimensional, became secure enough to share the part they played with their therapist, whether that part was simply to sing, to dance, to cry, to sulk, it was all in an effort to feel safe.

Meanwhile, Lynette was interested in identifying and meeting the alters, and to find out the part each had played in my circumstance of abuse. As she became more familiar with them, more memories began to surface. This was interesting, and associating them to the "noises" or commands each was making to me, was beginning to make sense. I realized that each little girl, although seemingly so simplistic, was complicated enough to want individual validation, hence each acting out in her own way.

But even more amazing to me was the fact that just as individuals who witness a common event often come away with their own distinct impression of what took place, so too did each of the alters, in this case the children. This difference in memory recall caused me a lot of anxiety as it was important to me to be able to sort, organize, understand them all, as if in doing so it would bring some sort of reason, some logic, some rationale to it all. The change or conflict of even the smallest detail would upset and confuse me, causing me to question my sanity and the validity of my memories. So, this time in counseling was particularly difficult. Often I would leave a session totally wrung out, tired and just wiped out from the work and strain of going back and reliving the ordeal of the memories. Each little girl, depending on her main function and type of her personality, colored the events. The Singer, the Dancer and the Player were happier, more optimistic, so they would tone down the negative emotions like fear and pain, trying their best to make everything all right. The Chrissies who were negative, such as the Crier and the Pouter, refused to see anything good or trustworthy.

At the very same time I was still leading the life of super mom: a Christian woman with two young sons, holding down a twenty-hour-per-week job, co-coordinating a large children's program in the church, leading a women's Bible study group, looking after a large acreage, and working tirelessly in my therapy to get better. It was daunting. No one knew my secret life of therapy and anguish. Of course my mood swings were often evident but no one really paid much mind to them because I had always been an emotional person. It was very important, I believed, to be busy and productive. I abided by the old rural saying: there is no problem that a hard day's work and a good meal won't fix.

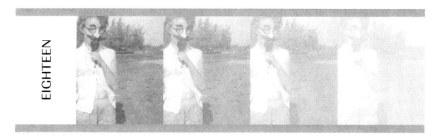

# EIGHTEEN

# *Chrissy*

Over the weeks in therapy, the children were able to freely express themselves. They felt comfortable with Lynette and she coaxed them out one by one. Perhaps because of that, this memory came together, and it was a glimpse into all of my alters.

It is a hot sunny day. Chrissy, a vibrant, energetic eight-year-old with pale blue eyes in a round freckled face, framed by an unruly mass of golden-red curls, is playing in the sand. It is what remains of the farmhouse that had been lost in a fire the year before. This is right across from the out-house that sits back just a little into a row of natural growth trees. Chrissy, who is always busy, always smiling, is deep into her digging in the warm sand. She hears the squeak of the screen door. She doesn't look up.

"Chrissy," she hears him say. Now she looks up and sees him point to the outhouse. Suddenly her head is a cacophony of noises and voices, all rushing in with their distinct personalities.

The Dark One and all the swirly ones—who are so far away and who swirl—begin yelling, "RUN!"

Suddenly she feels comforted as if the Kind Old Lady had wrapped her arms around her. It is her; the Kind Old

Lady then whispers to Chrissy, "Shush, and remember never run." She relaxes into the arms of the Kind Old Lady.

The Crier is now crying, but silently and without tears.

The Singer starts to croon quietly in her mind. The rest of the little girls love it when the Singer arrives. Today, she sings, "Clementine." Melodically she begins, "Oh my darling, oh my darling, oh my darling Clementine . . ."

Someone says, "It's time to go!" She rises robotically, showing no emotion. She walks stiff-legged, one foot in front of the other, like the march of the tin soldiers; like the last time, and the time before that, and the countless other times before that. Straight to the outhouse she marches. He doesn't need to tell her where to go; she knows this route.

The outhouse was what was referred to as a two-seater because of the two holes. She makes her way up between the holes onto the cold, rough plywood. She pushes herself back against the wall, as far back as she can. She hopes it will swallow her up, but it never does. It is smelly and dark and scary in here.

The Crier is still there, and she is being comforted by the Kind Old Lady, who again says "Shush. Shush, my sweetheart. I am here. I will hold you, and protect you. I am here."

The Singer is even more animated, performing other old favorite songs, "You are my sunshine, my only sunshine . . ." and now the Dancer is there doing a kind of Highland fling, a Celtic dance, with her toes pointed and her legs kicking high.

There are no crowds of people in this circus-like atmosphere. There is just one quiet little girl, huddled against the back wall of the toilet, shivering slightly.

The hazy swirlers—who have been whirling around in the background like crazy static on a radio, in and out, louder then softer, like a reoccurring buzz—are now silent.

The Dark One is silent. She worries about him because he can make Dad really mad. The Dark One will be the one to suddenly kick or bite, or be yelling at her to run, to hide, to tell. The rest know that kind of thing never works and almost always results in more terror.

She wonders what it will be today. Perhaps her mouth; it tastes yucky but hurts far less. She hopes there will be no blood. The door opens for a second and sunlight fills the outhouse. She squints. Then it is dark. He is so big. He blocks the sun. The door slams shut behind him and it is really dark.

The Crier is raising an awful fuss. The Crier tries to melt into the wall of the outhouse. She weeps then sobs. She has her head in her hands and her body is shaking.

The Dark One yells, he is furious, "RUN, KICK, SCREAM!" he shouts to all the children, but they are too scared to listen to him. In fact they just want him to be quiet.

The Kind Old Lady shushes the Dark One along with the Crier and the Singer. They must be quiet. She gathers the children in her arms and hugs tight. She releases for a minute then hugs tighter. Everyone is quiet, except for the Singer a long way in the distance.

Zzzzip. He is unzipping his pants. Look down, do not look up, never look up. Only he can say when to look up. He gets mad if you open your eyes or look up—and when that happens it will hurt them even more. It will be over soon. Chrissy is wearing shorts. He grabs her skinny, bare knees and pulls her away from the wall. He places his huge warm thing between her knees and he pushes her legs tight around it.

He's not taking her pants off. Yippee. He rubs himself back and forth, back and forth. He is moaning and it is soon over.

There is giggling and dancing. The Crier stops. It is okay. This is a "no pain" day. The Singer continues. The Dark One is gone, as is the static hum the swirlers create. They seem to appear in the beginning or middle of one of these times with Dad. They help everyone make believe that nothing bad is happening. Swirlers are unpredictable. We never know when they might arrive but when they do it is a noisy, distracting background buzz.

He didn't even get any of the yucky, messy sticky stuff on her clothes. Zzzip. He closes his zipper. Chrissy feels a pat on the head. "That's my good girl, remember to count," he says. The door opens and the toilet is momentarily flooded with sunlight again. He is gone. They always argue about how far to count—is fifty enough or should it be 100?

A few minutes later Chrissy emerges from the outhouse. It is warm and bright. The birds are signing. The air is fresh.

The little girl steps carefully into the sunlight. She scurries back to the sandbox. She digs and sings one of her favorite songs that she learned in school: "Oh my darling, oh my darling, oh my darling, Clementine . . ."

This had been a good day, a very good "no pain" day.

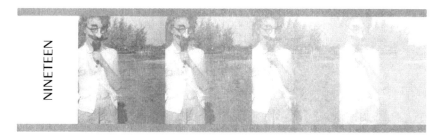

# NINETEEN

# Time in the Sun

To get to this stage in the therapy was a long haul. I would arrive at Lynette's office feeling calm, ready to start another chapter in my recovery process. I never knew what the sessions would hold in store. No matter how tough the appointments themselves were, Lynette and I usually spent a few minutes at the end just chatting, usually small talk. I imagine this was to settle the girls and me down. It was always a nice way to honor the children.

"Have a chair, Chris." Lynette would say, "How has your week been?" Chris was the name I used at this time, all my friends and family called me Chris even though Christine was my given name.

The majority of the time I would respond, "It's been a good week."

"May we start with prayer?" she would ask. She always started with an opening prayer but always asked permission first.

"Of course, I would love that," I'd answer.

"Right," someone in my head is saying sarcastically, "Love that . . . please, this is junk, and you don't need this!"

Crying started. If the sad little girl was appearing, the session would almost inevitably start with outward crying.

Lynette began the opening prayer: "Dear Lord, please watch

over us and protect us with your eternal love. Offer Chris and the children peace and strength to get through today's session and in the healing time to come."

I didn't want any of the kids to appear, *please God keep them away today.* Lynette and I had named them all "Chrissy" because we felt that they were different modes of the same alter or personality. I didn't want any of those Chrissies to be here: not the Singer, or the Dancer, or the Crier—none of them. I didn't want any of the little girls to be here. I didn't always feel this way; sometimes denying their existence just seemed easier and this was one of those times.

Accepting the reality of multiple personalities and the reason for their creation had been a formidable task. Reaching inward and further and accepting the many alters, acknowledging the repeated abuse that created these little girls, was a cruel nightmare to have to live through again. As difficult and gut-wrenching as this was, I was determined to slug through this ordeal. I was going to help them, just as they had helped me. They had shaken me into recognizing the abuse that had been part of our collective childhood, the one I had buried for decades. It was time for them to rest, to find peace. Now I needed to find a way to heal them—so that I could heal, and move on.

Each of the little girls was almost one-dimensional: the Giggler, the Dancer, the Crier, the Singer. And even though the body—my body—had grown up, these little girls had not; they remained children. They all remained in my mind as looking like young Chrissy, with the unruly mop of curly hair. Physically, they all looked the same; the difference was their behavior and accompanying expressions. When they had their time and felt safe in therapy, they came one at a time, to sing, dance, cry, and giggle—whatever they had been created to do.

Lynette described the little girls to me as she met them in therapy. Sometimes this would happen at the end of a session. Occasionally I would ask at the end if I didn't remember meeting them during therapy. At other times Lynette would begin a session by recounting the previous one and how it went. Still other times I would have recall so we didn't have to rehash anything. She related how there was the Giggler, the Dancer, the Crier, and the Singer. They all seemed to have a clear idea of what their job was. Lynette talked about how important they had all been, each with their own separate jobs. They fulfilled their function and not much more or less. One thing was certain though, they all needed to be accepted individually, told how they were loved and needed as part of the whole. "Chris, I'd like you to go home this week and write each of the girls a letter. Tell them how they helped you and let them know how much you appreciate them. Bring them with you when we next meet."

Writing these letters was surreal and often I wondered what good it would do. There was seldom any emotion attached to the actual writing but when we shared them in Lynette's office many things could happen. Depending on which little girl was there: sadness and crying; fear to the point of shaking; laughter and joy when the Dancer and Giggler arrived; or confusion as it seemed they all wanted to talk at once. The letters were all basically the same and some written to more than one of the children at a time. They read like this:

Dearest Chrissy:

I am so grateful I have been able to talk to you recently. I knew you were there and I am sorry I never said anything before. I know you helped me through some bad, bad times, I am especially glad when I think of your singing. I loved your singing, it was so nice.

When our session was nearing an end that day Lynette said, "When you read that letter to Chrissy the Singer, you—the Chrissy alter—quit reading, got off the chair and sat on the floor in the corner and began to sing 'My Darling Clementine' and 'You Are My Sunshine.' " I did not remember this and when I first learned that I did this I felt a little embarrassed and silly. After all, I was a grown woman.

Lynette continued, "The same thing happened when you read

the letter to Chrissy the Dancer. She got up and danced a lively jig, pretending to be a Scottish dancer."

The letter-reading session with Chrissy the Crier had taken nearly two hours. When I read to her she grabbed a soft pillow and cowered in the corner sobbing. Lynette held her, consoling her and trying to bring her back to center. Toward the end of the session she had even gotten Chrissy the Crier to play a little with some pretty colored building blocks.

"In order to integrate these personalities, Chris," Lynette told me, "We're going to have to give each one their time in the sun, so to speak. This is why I asked you to write each of them a letter.

As I brought the letters to the therapy sessions and read them out loud Lynette would tell each of the child alters how special their job had been and how thankful we all were that they had been there for me. Lynette was able to talk directly with some, some she held, some she played with and others were more timid and took more time and reassurance.

I would visualize going back and bringing them to a safe place with me. It was many hours of hard work with Lynette leading the way. Occasionally this would get unsettling for Lynette and she would phone the therapist who had agreed to act as a consultant through the process.

Slowly but surely, over a period of about eight months, the alters began to distinguish themselves from one another. Then a gentle blending took place as one by one the Chrissies were not there anymore.

This process did however threaten and stir up some very disturbing emotions. On a couple of occasions Lynette had noticed that after one or more of the children had been in therapy I would appear agitated and angry. This happened just before I would leave a session, and for that reason Lynette had chosen not to address this, fearing I would go home upset.

Finally this angry person did arrive at a therapy session and it was a very unsettling occurrence for Lynette and me. Lynette said, "This was a difficult day and I don't know that I handled it the best way. I feel like we are getting into deeper water, and that I might be getting in over my head. We made a deal that I would continue to work with you, with outside assistance, and I am going to honor that agreement. However, I must be honest with you, having someone with more expertise in this area would greatly benefit your healing process. I strongly recommend that we bring someone else on board."

I sat there stunned, not knowing how to answer.

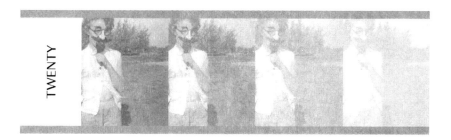

# TWENTY

# *What's My Line?*

Christine was my given name, ironically chosen by my dad, but it didn't stick. From a very young age everyone around me called me Chris, except for my older aunts and grandparents who called me Chrissy. However as I grew older they began to call me Chris as well.

As the therapy with Lynette progressed I was often overwhelmed with emotion. Unearthing all this long-buried horror was a Pandora's box. While I needed to know the truth and the examination of my childhood was key to my healing, reliving the torment was often like opening a container of spoiled meat in your refrigerator: the minute you lift up the lid you are overcome with the sights and the smells. While in the midst of this, I began to hear another voice in my head. It was stronger and said things to me like: *"We can do this. Let me help!"* or *"Don't buckle under now—we can handle anything."* This voice—a woman's voice—was calm and authoritative. I liked her. She made me feel safe and in control. To me the name Christine had an innate strength and many times I wished people would call me that instead of Chris, and so this voice in my head became Christine.

I suppose I had always heard the voice of Christine—as well as the other voices—at some point or another. Since I hadn't known any differently, I thought this was normal. After I started in psychotherapy and was diagnosed with DID these adult voices, or alters, moved to the forefront and became more active. It was during therapy that I learned of their roles in my life and I established their names.

"These identities formed ultimately to protect you," explained Lynette. "As the abuse happened to you and you were powerless to stop it you dissociated, or split. You went out of your body. This is why you had all the children, all the manifestations of Chrissy: the one who danced to escape the horror; the one who sang through the molestation to drown out the horrible sounds; the ones who swirled were there to distract you; and the one who cried to let out all the sadness when you could not be seen crying. As you got older," she continued, "the personalities changed and evolved."

I learned that my alters were not just odd personalities who formed haphazardly and acted willy-nilly. Instead they were a *system* of people who offered opinions and took action in my life:

*Elizabeth* is a kind protector—a.k.a., the Kind Old Lady—and offers intuitional nudges at every opportunity. She holds all the memories. She is very feminine yet also very strong. She is like Great- Grandma Annie and is spiritual, wise and non-judgmental.

*Sally* is just plain fun. A party girl, she is very sexual, passionate and somewhat immature. She is very feminine and drinks to have fun. She was the one who had sex with my dad—that was her job. It was also Sally who jumped into the back seats of cars with any boy who asked when I was a teenager.

*John* is the dark, angry protector who occasionally yells warnings to the others and often wreaks havoc. He hates weakness and comes to a point where he cannot, will not, tolerate what he perceives as abuse—which comes to mean even the slightest amount of disrespect. For this, he seeks revenge and considers himself entitled. He is asexual, an atheist, and sees drinking as a huge weakness. John, along with Elizabeth, holds all the memories. Together, he and Elizabeth kept those memories from the others.

*Chris* is a caretaker and all things maternal. She is the consummate "cookie baker" and gentle church mom. She sees the bright side of everything, or tries to. She loves to laugh, to enjoy life, and loves nature and bright colors. A loyal friend, she is honest and faithful and the first one to volunteer when someone needs help. However, she holds the guilt and drinks to self-medicate, to escape not feeling good enough.

*Christine* is the empowered, managerial, take-charge organizer. She is efficient, unemotional, intellectual, agnostic, asexual and a non-drinker. This well-spoken woman is not intimidated by anyone. She empathizes with Chris and her role as a mom, but has little tolerance for her people- pleasing tendencies.

❦

Therapy was kind of like the old game show *What's My Line?* You never knew who might emerge on any given day. Neither Lynette, nor I, had any idea how my time in therapy—and my life—would be thrown into a tailspin. It all happened with the bold emergence of the angry one, the Dark One, the one who called himself John.

He came into Lynette's office one day, not long after she had told me again that she felt unable to appropriately handle the place in therapy we had arrived at now. Walking purposefully into the office, he took a wallet out of his pocket, and scribbled in the checkbook. With hardly so much as a glance at Lynette, he threw a check on her desk.

"I have had enough of this 'do-good' bullshit therapy," he said. "I have listened to enough fucking crying about all the crap in the past, it's time to move on, get a fucking life. You're paid in full now, so I won't be wasting my time or yours over this anymore." He was on his feet and going toward the door.

"Before you go," Lynette said, "I would like to hear more from you, and could I talk to Chris before you go?" He hesitated only a few seconds before pounding out the door, once more giving it a big slam.

This was the dark, angry man's first emergence in defense of himself, where he would first acknowledge—if not so much in words than in actions—how he was feeling threatened by the therapy process.

I was back in the car, my knees were shaking, and all I could do was cry. I heard an irritated voice in my head saying, "No, fucking way they are getting rid of me like they are doing with the kids."

My recollection of this session was sketchy, I just felt scared. I had learned at a very early age to avoid conflict at any cost. When the Dark One spoke to me he was always angry, always tearing someone apart, pointing out how I was still being abused.

Once I arrived safely home I called Lynette to get the details. I was very upset and frightened. I was afraid of John, I knew he was capable of bad things—he was always stealing and lying, and getting me into trouble, like the time he had slid the blade of one of his ice skates over a fellow classmate's head in grade five. John claimed it had been all an accident, he hadn't meant it, this boy was sitting on the bottom step, he just happened to walk by with his skates over his arm. There was blood all over the place and the boy required over twelve stitches. The teacher bought John's story: it was an accident. In truth, the boy had sent Chris a filthy note asking her if she would like to "fuck him"—and it had angered John to take revenge.

I was very upset by this session and John's appearance at it, and so I wrote the following letter to Lynette that day:

Dear Lynette:

The appearance of John, (the kids called him the Black One or the Angry One, before we came to know him as John—it had nothing to do with skin color, more to do with a child's understanding of good and evil, like in Western movies; the good guys always wore white hats and the bad guys black hats) at your office recently was as unsettling to me as it was to you. It has, however, prompted some serious reflection on my state of affairs.

I have decided to "settle" for things as they are. Oh, I have entertained great dreams of university degrees, helping other incest victims and so on, but the fact remains that dealing with the everyday is about all I can handle. To strive for normality or to think I can attain such lofty heights has become a form of abuse in itself.

I have a husband and children who love me; my church, friends, fellow workers and employer respect me. I know that often they deserve better than they get from me. In many ways I feel inadequate. This time in therapy, even this time figuring out about the abuse, makes me wonder: what possible good is this doing my children? What parent can really say any different; don't we all feel like we are falling short? I have learned many things in the past three years. I understand (at least in part) how the incest has scared me to the very fiber of my soul. I have placed the responsibility of the abuse on my abuser and I accept no part in it.

I do accept responsibility in my healing process and understand it to be a lifelong process. I accept the formation of dissociative identity disorder as a means of survival. I have accomplished a sort of integration (more a cooperation) between Chris and Christine; these two leaders will continue to identify, accept and love the others. To what extent full integration of the other three will be achieved is not a priority. Of course there is John, the angry man you just met and he is powerful. I fear his actions, but believe as I prove to him how valuable he is to us he will join me just as the other "children" have.

I alone will deal with this, no one else will ever really get close enough to understand and besides no one who is close to me now will ever have what it takes to truly hang in there. Even though I know why the dissociative identity disorder happened and live with it every day, it reaches past my conscience to a level of reality that no one should ever have to know exists. Exist it does!

So my reality as I see it is this: I have a family and friends who love and respect me. I have a God who truly loves me and will always be there, who I don't have to explain any of this to. I have a job I enjoy and do well. I am active (not overactive) in my church and in my community.

I maintain a warm, inviting home and all that that entails (doctor appointments, dentist, youth group, kids' club, paying bills, laundry, cooking, cleaning, baking, and so on). I plan birthdays, anniversaries, and even the odd Tupperware party. I watch ball games, school plays, science fairs, and sports meets. I love going to auction sales, yard sales and crocheting. I enjoy reading, music and hilarious movies. I enjoy going for rides with my husband, wrestling with the kids and listening to them pray. I enjoy my computer and flower arranging and I take time for close friends and myself.

Sometimes I get tired and yell at the kids and I'm not as nice as I should be. What mom is?

Sex is still a roller-coaster ride, sometimes thrilling and wonderful, sometimes scary, sometimes boring, sometimes nonexistent but I continue to work at it. When you read all this over, it really isn't so bad. Is it?

I am reminded of the concern I had upon realizing my multiplicity that I would not be able to function. Well, I believe I am functioning quite well. Oh, certainly not with the peace and single-mindedness than non-DID's have but fulfilling all my obligations just the same.

I will continue to journal and work in the *Wounded Heart* book. I will cancel further appointments with you, for now at least. I will attempt to achieve a peaceful coexistence among my alters. You seem to pose a threat to that right now. You no doubt will be seeing me in the future as this probably won't work, but I have to try and like I mentioned earlier in my letter anything else feels like more abuse.

Sincerely and with much gratitude,

Chris

---

I didn't see Lynette for three months. During that time I allowed myself to slip back into almost a state of semi-denial. I never tried to deny the sexual abuse had occurred, but I did try to convince myself that the actual damage done was minimal. I also determined once again that the answer was that I just had to live a fuller Christian life. That had to be the answer and so I threw myself even deeper into the church: more prayer, more Bible study, more, more and more. It should have been paying off with more peace and contentment but it wasn't. What it was doing was bringing me more recognition as a very active, capable, charismatic leader. However, I still sometimes woke up during the night scared to death and the flashbacks and terror of being in my own yard still haunted me. Following God's handbook wasn't working. I felt like a complete failure, a total hypocrite. A voice in my head kept saying: "Don't let these people fool you, they are not what they appear." The inner turmoil was rising, so soon I was back in therapy—and back to my family physician who saw no problem with prescribing pills to help me with anxiety and get better sleep. The drug worked initially but seldom took me through the whole night, and the longer I took it the more I needed to get any effect at all.

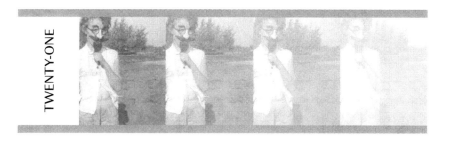

# TWENTY-ONE

# The Dark, Angry One Emerges

I needed to know more about the very angry Dark One. He had made it clear, however, that he did not want to be referred to by this description. During one of his tirades he said, "Don't call me that. My name is not 'the Dark One'. My name is John."

Who was he, and where had he gotten his name? Pondering this question, I remembered a relative named John—my father's great-uncle—who was somewhat dour, never smiled, and always seemed surrounded by a sense of foreboding. Perhaps my alter John was named after him. Uncle John lived in my grandparents' yard in a one-room shack way back in the woods. He lived alone—unless you counted the large feral cat colony that surrounded him. The long, narrow path to his house was surrounded by thick bushes but when you got close to his home you were rewarded with plum trees. The fruit had thick, bitter skin, but the inside was tender and sweet. I would bite through and suck the sweet center out. It seemed like a very long walk to his home and the trees were very tall but I never felt afraid. Since the cats were wild, they would scurry away as I approached, never letting me pet them.

Inside Uncle John's shack was a huge wood cook stove on one wall and a table and four chairs in the middle of the room. Against the other wall was a small cot, covered with thick, grey wool blankets that were cloaked in cat hair. I would sit at the kitchen table and look around. Uncle John seemed so old. He always wore the same heavy, brown tweed coat and a felt hat. He never spoke much. In fact, I couldn't recall him speaking at all. Someone told me that he was from France so I assumed at the time that all French people were uncommunicative.

The visits always ended the same. It was my favorite part. On the way out the door he would give me Smith Brothers licorice-flavored cough drops. He always gave me two, each one wrapped in white crinkly paper. I would pop one in my mouth right away and place the other one in my pocket for later. I loved how the licorice smelled and, even better, how it tasted. I especially loved how smooth the drops felt as they dissolved in my mouth.

I couldn't remember seeing Uncle John outside his shack— until Grandpa and Grandma received electricity. This monumental event was soon followed by another: the arrival of a television. This led to a new family tradition: Saturday night hockey.

The whole family would be there, but Uncle John held sway over the evening. The routine was always the same. He would walk onto the porch, take off his felt hat, and lay it on the cupboard by the water pail. Then he would proceed into the living room and sit in Grandpa's chair, a wonderful ornately carved wooden rocker. Uncle John was the only person other than Grandpa who ever sat in the chair. The TV reception was poor at best, looking more like a black and white snowstorm. Still, everyone sat glued to the screen. We cheered for any team but the Montreal Canadiens. Those people did not speak proper French, according to Grandfather. You could never tell whom Uncle John cheered for since he wore the same expression through the whole game. After the game, Grandma served coffee and snacks at the kitchen table. Uncle John would get up, put on his hat, and give us kids another wonderful licorice flavored cough drop on his way out the door. He'd disappear into the night.

Was Uncle John the inception for my alter John? He was strong, respected and somewhat feared by our whole family. Who knows? This was speculation at best, but everything in some strange way ties itself to another. One thing for sure, Uncle John was never as angry as my alter John.

⚜

My first vivid recollection of John's existence surfaced with the memory of Larry the neighbor boy.

*"STOP THIS!"* an enraged man had yelled, but it hadn't been Dad and he was the only adult male there. This anger scared me and I wanted him to go away. The children were especially frightened by his deep, bellowing voice. They were scared he would say something to Dad and then I would get a bad beating, we were all sure of it.

I learned in counseling that each alter served a specific purpose. Lynette told me this about John: "He holds the anger, the pain, the resentment, the hatred, every negative thought or emotion connected to the abuse had been his property." It was as though he remembered every lasting detail of those horrific memories. That was his job. In counseling, the memories of the abuse surfaced and John was more than ready to "tell." When the memories revealed themselves and came tumbling out of my mouth, John spewed them out, spit them out, with all the anger he could muster. And he didn't limit his opinions to the sexual abuse in childhood. He had more than plenty to say about what he considered my taking "abuse," be it emotional or physical, with the men who passed my way, including Rick. It seemed that John hated men—or at least many of the men who had been in my life.

Not that his hatred was only focused on men. He abhorred any disrespect anyone showed to me and he would constantly berate me for allowing it to happen. The good side of John was that he was fiercely loyal to me. He didn't want anyone to give me any shit of any nature. The downside was that as a strong and virile male, he was ready to do battle with anyone and everyone. Unfortunately the price for his protection in my adult life would be very high.

John especially hated anything sexually inappropriate, but as long as I was able to protect myself or counter it he remained silent. I suspect that in the early years of my promiscuity, because I had wanted the sexual involvement with the many high school boys, John remained silent. It was as though he understood I was a willing participant, and in fact, the instigator at times. I realized in therapy, however, that the willing participant was really Sally.

When I think back to all the noises and voices in my head, in those times when John remained silent, he was allowing the other alters to be themselves—he let them "do their job" of protecting me or informing me in their own special way. The system of alters ran like the board of directors of a corporation. Each alter had a specific function and they all reported to me, the CEO.

Things started to change, however, the more I got into therapy and the more I excavated and analyzed. John was especially angry about the way Chris, my maternal caretaker, was used and disrespected by my husband. Rick's affair was inexcusable; still I should have seen it coming. Rick's general attitude toward women was always bad and that would never change. He considered women lesser beings, constantly joked about how stupid they were and enjoyed putting me down, especially in front of others. Perhaps that was learned behavior; in his family his mom's only important purpose was having babies, cooking and cleaning—woman's work, which they did not consider "real" work.

While "the system" paid little to no attention to the dynamics between my husband and myself, and while I settled for the relationship Rick and I had, it upset John to no end. In fact it seemed the harder he tried to make me see how poorly I was being treated by Rick, the more I ran around singing my spouse's praises, telling everyone what a great husband I had. I had even told Lynette how wonderful and supportive he was, and this made John livid.

"If he is a great husband I am the bloody King of England!" screamed John. "Have you forgotten the AFFAIR? He was out screwing around, drinking and having fun while you were home holding it all together. Did he ever think of you? No! Did he think about the kids? No! He was too busy getting laid. You think that's going to change? Hah! You are really naive, Chris. Wake up and smell the coffee, sister!"

This was the beginning of a whole new formation among the alters—everyone was going to be heard. No longer were John and Elizabeth the only ones holding the memories and no longer were Chris and Christine the only ones organizing and running the show.

My marriage seemed to be the project up for discussion among my alters: what I would now refer to collectively as my Board or the Directors. Rick's affair was really the beginning of the end of our relationship but the alters stirred the pot and hastened its demise.

John would harass me: "How can you be so dumb? Open your eyes, or don't, it's only a matter of time till this asshole shows his true colors." His angry voice continually cursed Rick in my mind.

Elizabeth did her best to quiet and comfort: "John, shush, you are not helping."

Chris cried; she was confused and unable to deal with Rick's sarcasm, dismissive attitude and the thought that he might have another affair.

Christine, the efficient manager, tried to handle everything. The issue, however, was not simply Rick's bad husband skills but also the unfinished business of my horrendous childhood.

Lynette had told me, "Your inner children were deeply wounded, and this craziness in your life will continue until they are healed, and only then can the adults heal. There is so much more work to be done."

John was livid. "No more!" he shouted. "No more!"

The Directors were mostly in favor of Chris continuing to work on her marriage, for the sake of the children. The instinct to mother and protect Craig and Cory had overpowered John's anger, but only temporarily. It was the beginning of John's assault on the world. John's retribution had begun. He needed to be in charge or the abuse, as he saw it, would continue. Disrespect, after all, equaled abuse.

"You are all pathetic. Get your fucking heads out of the sand!" he would shout in the middle of a quiet day, scaring me half to death. He would pop in at inopportune times, like in the middle of intimacy. With John whirling through my head like a tornado, I could hardly stand to be touched by Rick and would avoid sex altogether because it was just too awful an experience.

John was very clever and determined to break my husband and me apart. He knew that if I was ever going to leave Rick, I would have to remember more of my horrendous past. So he started his crusade of releasing the sordid details of those memories and making my adult life a chaotic mess.

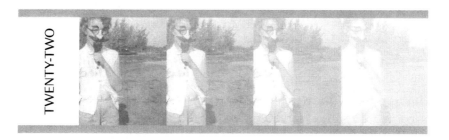

TWENTY-TWO

# Entitlement and Revenge

I tried my best to control John. I was not ready to give in to his demands to get rid of Rick and so I had to devise a way to tune him out. One strategy was to get even busier than I was already. I buried myself in work and projects. I got a job with a home care agency and went back to school to get my home care special care aide certificate. I also took on another cause: I became president of the local chapter of PRIDE (Parents' Resource Institute on Drug Education).

I was back to seeing Lynette on a regular basis. I was relieved that she was still my therapist. We decided to focus the therapy strictly on healing the effects of the sexual abuse. I continued working through the book *The Wounded Heart* by Dr. Dan Allender. Also, I attended a group therapy session that Lynette had established for women who had been sexually abused. I don't know if any of the other participants had DID or not—I doubted it—but it felt right for me to be among women with similar childhood experiences. The four of us met once every two weeks and each had individual sessions during the other week. I found our group encounters very interesting and enjoyed meeting and getting to know others who had been abused. We were all about the same age, and were all married with children. I found it remarkable that these women who had been so damaged as children could appear so "together." All of us were impeccably dressed, never a hair out of place. We had all been programmed to look good; it was all about keeping the secret and we all believed that no one was going to believe us if we did tell.

Therapy, prayer, work, the church, volunteering, the acreage, the children, and lots and lots of Valium helped me through the days and nights. Still, yard work was becoming more and more frightening, as I never knew when the memories would hit. Looking after the huge garden and yard was no longer a joy. I began to insist we move to town. Rick was working away from home anyway, so it really made sense for us to be in an urban area.

Not long after I came to this conclusion, we moved out of the house and back into town. I figured that maybe moving out of my childhood home would stop my mental torment. Much to my horror, nothing really changed—at least not with the alters. John had his own relentless agenda to plant seeds of distrust by pointing out even the slightest insult against me from other people, particularly from Rick. He trusted no one and seemed to blame everyone; he thought the other alters needed to quit being so soft. He also thought himself smarter then most and didn't tolerate what he deemed stupidity from the other alters and people in general.

I had received my certificate in home care and loved the people I worked for. John, however, viewed my clients as just more users: people in a world of the ungrateful with their own hidden agendas.

Our financial situation was pretty grim, and John saw the cause as massive stupidity on my husband's part. "If he hadn't been drinking and carousing you wouldn't have this problem," he barked. Just about this time I acquired a client named Mrs. McClaren. She had been my second-grade teacher, which was also a time when some of my worst sexual abuse episodes had taken place. More ironic than that was the fact that she was the wife of our family doctor. As a child I was constantly at his office—and not just for colds and ear aches. I had chronic throat infections and vaginal infections long before I ever reached puberty. Looking back on this as an adult, I know that Dr. McClaren should have questioned this. If he had not known outright, he should have at least been suspicious; there was only one reason why these things were happening. It was just one more missed opportunity to save a child.

Dr. McClaren had long since died. While he left Mrs. McClaren in good financial shape, dementia had robbed her of the ability to live independently. On my five-day-a-week visits to her house I listened to the same loop over and over again. "You know I was a teacher," she would say. "I was a kind, wonderful teacher and all the children loved me and I loved them." Or she would play the loop about her husband, "My husband was such a wonderful doctor. Everyone in town looked up to him; he saved so many lives."

This unnerved John to no end. "A good doctor my ass!" he'd say. "He knew what was happening. He was just a lazy coward. He let that scumbag keep on with his filth while children suffered. Maybe he can't pay for his sins but this old bitch wife of his can!"

Part of Mrs. McClaren's care involved handling some of her daily financial affairs: taking her grocery shopping, helping her pay bills and taking her to the bank. Her children lived quite a distance and they felt comfortable with this arrangement.

Mrs. McClaren had never needed to scrimp and save. She was used to having a lot of money and kept a couple hundred dollars in her purse at all times. The ready cash was too much of a temptation for John. At first it was fifty dollars once in awhile. He had no remorse about taking the money from her; in fact he loved the feeling. The combination of entitlement and revenge was a total turn-on for him. But soon this small-time thievery wasn't enough and it only fueled his ego and lust for more. He was hell-bent on getting even with the McClaren's for turning a blind eye to my childhood abuse. He began to plot his first major theft.

I fought furiously at first. We would argue sometimes, "This is wrong, this can land us in jail!" Mostly the strategy was to divert John's attention by good deeds and working harder, staying busy, busy, busy. But eventually I had little left to fight with. I was not at the head of the Board of Directors anymore—it was more like the

Directors of the Board, with the CEO sitting on the sidelines like some kind of figurehead. I remained the supermom, church volunteer, even the one who showed up for therapy, but seldom had memory of any of it and often came home from work not remembering being there. My weight skyrocketed to an all-time high, and I put on nearly fifty pounds in one year. Occasionally I would be aware of the stealing and was sick about it, but that just added to the depression and feeling of being a complete failure. I was losing the battle. John was running the show. It was Valium and food for me; I felt totally out of control.

In my "absence" John had gotten access to Mrs. McClaren's bank accounts. He borrowed enough of her identification to open an account, and went to a neighboring town some sixty miles away to set up his scam. He had already opened a post office box there using her name. The only other alter who had any knowledge of this was Christine and she really didn't care one way or another. John was on a major power trip and got a big charge as he announced to the bank representative, "I am a retired teacher and am moving here to be closer to my children and grandchildren."

"How nice," said the banker as she typed up the account card. It went off without a hitch. He mustered all the charm and composure of Christine and was so convincing to the clerk that she didn't notice the nearly thirty-year difference between his and Mrs. McClaren's age on the documentation. He walked out with a bank account and a credit card.

On the way home I stopped and threw up on the side of the road. I didn't know why I was sick; after all I had spent the morning shopping and had a nice lunch out, hadn't I?

Over the next eighteen months John would transfer over ten thousand dollars from Mrs. McClaren's real account into that bank account. He also spent nearly four thousand dollars on the credit card, then made the necessary payments on the card from the stolen money in the fraudulent account.

Elizabeth chastised me for this, "What is happening? Stop the stealing. It is wrong and you will get caught." She also questioned my decision to move off the family farm, "The children loved the farm. It was perfect for them. Why did you leave?"

I did feel guilty about moving the boys off the farm, and the stealing, but I had been granted a bit of a reprieve from the abuse flashbacks since the move into town. As far as John, for the most part I wasn't putting up a huge fight against him. I just didn't have it in me and I had to admit that when John pushed me I enjoyed spending the money on my family. I purchased a two-car garage and a trip to Florida to celebrate my twenty-fifth wedding anniversary. That pissed John off to no end. Hubby benefitting from "his" money was *not* part of the plan. The Florida trip was completely inexplicable to everyone; none of the board even liked Rick much, let alone loved him anymore, and here we were paying for a vacation.

I had virtually no control over the stealing and didn't remember doing it, but occasionally when John was in the middle of something I would become aware and try to undo the damage by returning money. On one particular occasion, John had withdrawn one thousand dollars from the account. I was half way home when suddenly I was aware of what was happening. I turned the car around and replaced the money, not just into the "fake" account but right back into Mrs. McClaren's account. That happened a couple of times over the eighteen-month period—and luckily for me later on, the paper trail would help substantiate dissociative identity disorder.

Shortly after the move to town I was faced with another dilemma. My longtime therapist and lifeline to sanity, Lynette, was quitting. While she had tried to do this many times before I had always convinced her that I needed her. Now there was no chance I could persuade her to stay. "This is very difficult for me to do," said Lynette. "I am closing my practice because I am starting a family. It wouldn't be fair to my patients, nor to my children, if I stayed on. In God's name I promise you that I will place you in good hands. I owe that to you," she said.

While I understood her decision it was very upsetting nonetheless. I had come to count on the sessions with her, even though I was too ashamed and frightened to share about John's activity. I had been attending sessions regularly again after the three-month layoff and it gave me hope that things could and would get better but only if I worked at it. I tried to see another therapist in the same office. He had joined Lynette in a few sessions with me before she quit and initially I thought it would work. I soon realized, however, that without Lynette's presence this was not a good fit—there was no chemistry at all—so I stopped treatment altogether while I went looking for another therapist.

"Dear God, please help me," I said on bended knees. But no amount of prayer seemed to help. I was guilty, depressed and fat. For so long my faith in God had helped sustain me, but now I was losing it. I had so many questions, including: How could a "good" God allow something as evil as child abuse? Where was God then? Where is God now? God had forsaken me, and I started to forsake him: I sought solace in pills, taking more of them in a stronger dosage.

Without Lynette's help, I felt lost again. I tried a couple of other therapists in my home community but once they discovered my diagnosis and realized how long and complicated my treatment would be, they refused to accept me as a patient. More than once I heard the line, "I wish that it could be otherwise, but I just do not have the qualifications to deal with your case." Those who would accept me gave me "bad vibes" and so I crossed them off my list.

It was actually the last doctor on my list of rejections who tossed me a lifeline that would prove to be a godsend. "While I am not qualified to handle your case, I do know someone who is: Dr. Douglas Jurgens," she said as she scribbled down his phone number for me. It was a strange and fortuitous coincidence, indeed, for Dr. Jurgens was the psychologist who Lynette had sought out as a consultant when she felt overwhelmed by the complications of my treatment. I had never met him, and was unaware of his presence during my treatment as he was on speakerphone, and I was often oblivious to what was happening in the room at the time. I had no idea who he was when I first met him and he did not reveal to me for some time that he was already familiar with my case.

We hit it off right away, strangely enough. I say this because he was a large man and none of us were typically comfortable with that. He also wasn't what I would have deemed a conventional-looking therapist. He was twelve years younger than I was and had long hair, usually in a ponytail. I had thought that someone with the credentials to handle my complicated condition would need to be at least twelve years older than I was, sporting a short haircut, and wearing a stuffy tweed jacket with elbow patches. I should have learned my lesson with Lynette about not judging a book by its cover. This professional relationship proved to be an interesting, positive and life-changing partnership.

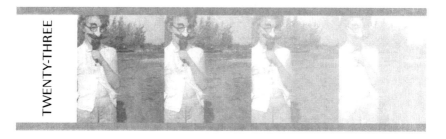

# TWENTY-THREE

# The Church Board versus My Board

I loved the church and everything it stood for. I had poured my heart and soul into it, working tirelessly in a variety of programs. I coordinated the Children's Club program for several years. It was one of the most effective community outreach programs the church had ever had, drawing in over sixty children. I spent hours developing new and innovative ways to teach the kids about the love of God. I was passionate about every detail.

The church gave me a lifeline through all the disappointment in my marriage, led me to find Lynette, and helped—at least at first—deal with the reality of my childhood and the discovery that I had DID. But then things started to change.

One of the pillars of the church community was a family I had modeled my life on. The husband and wife ran the local Christian bookstore, and they held the Wednesday night Bible study in their home. Their son and daughter were involved in the youth group, which the parents ran. Generous to a fault, they always gave of their time, money and attention. They were the ideal Christian family, everything I aspired to be, and everything I wished my family was.

Then I started noticing things that gave me a strange feeling in my gut. I saw the father put his hand on the small of his fourteen-year-old daughter's back one Sunday. Something about the way he let it linger there was just not right—it was more the way a husband might behave with his spouse, not his child. During our adult Bible studies held in their home, the girl would often sit in her Dad's lap, sometimes whispering in his ear, both of them giggling. Then the daughter started having "fainting spells" in church. Rather than seek medical attention, the father would take her out, missing Sunday school.

"Don't you get this?" John shouted, "It's bad, you know it's bad. Daddy is doing his daughter and you know it." John shouted the accusations but I blocked them. Not long after this, however, rumors circulated, which were eventually substantiated, that the daughter had an abortion.

The Directors flew into a frenzy. John ranted, "What did I tell you? What the hell did I tell you? Now will you finally listen to me?"

"John, please just shush!" implored Elizabeth desperately.

Chris just wanted all the noise to stop; conflict was the last thing she wanted. Finally, Christine arrived and a wave of calm descended, she said, "Stop it! This isn't going to accomplish anything. If we want to help this kid this nonsense has to stop!"

John was right about the issue but Christine was right about taking charge in a rational manner. I knew that I needed to do something to rescue the young girl who was obviously being mistreated under the guise of her loving, "pious" daddy. I did some investigation and was shocked to find out that there had been complaints against the father about inappropriate behavior with girls in the youth group. To my disgust it had been swept under the rug. Fear of confrontation nearly stopped me from doing anything about this situation, but my fear was counterbalanced by John's determination to get this girl some help. While he was not the compassionate type he recognized the similarities in this family and mine and he knew that I would never forgive myself if I didn't try to do something.

Christine systematically took charge. She made three phone

calls: one to the pastor, one to the assistant pastor, and one to the chairman of the church board. She demanded that they take action by first removing the couple from the youth group leadership and next by reporting the incidents to the local police.

The church board called an emergency meeting on a Monday night. They asked the couple to step down, at least temporarily, while the matter was further investigated. By the following Thursday the family had packed all their belongings and moved an entire province away. They said that they were unjustly accused and that they had no other recourse. They said if they could not do the work the Lord was calling them to do in this church, then they had to leave.

"Right!" John chided "And we are going to believe this garbage? What a load of crap!" Once more John was on a rant. He would not leave me alone. He knew the church was not going to handle this. He was furious.

Christine took over again and made the call to the Royal Canadian Mounted Police and soon an officer was out to talk to me. As it turned out it had not been the first time this perfect church family had been brought to their attention, but they needed more than speculation, which is what they already had been given by someone else. They did promise to consult the daughter who was now fifteen years old. Still, since she was a minor, the law stipulated that the parents must give their consent to let the police talk to her—unless she was the one who initiated contact with them.

John was pleased—he didn't have to say a word but he just exuded this air of smugness. He had the chink in the Christian wall that he wanted. He had been sizing up these so-called "good" folks for some time and he wasn't buying their façade.

I, on the other hand, continued the good Christian fight, attending church, and taking over the Wednesday night Bible study since the regular teachers had left the province. I still lead the children's club, and also helped form a young Christian women's group. I kept up my daily reading of the Scriptures and prayed more and more. I was so efficient and so charismatic that I became the first woman ever to be elected to the church board. This was quite a feat, really, because only two decades earlier this church had not even allowed women to vote in their meetings! This gave my sagging self-esteem a real boost.

Following closely on the heels of my election to the board came another groundbreaking development in my Christian life. The church I belonged to had a provincial conference of 120 churches. Some felt that the provincial conference had drifted away from the local church's needs. So, at one of the assemblies a six-member task force was formed to conduct a study on the grassroots concerns of its membership and to assess the local churches' strengths, weaknesses and needs. They also wanted to get a fair representation from who was attending their churches and suggestions on how better to serve them.

I was honored to be appointed to the task force, and represented the members who had no ethnic ties and were converts. I was assigned a number of churches. I brainstormed with them, then took my findings to the task force where we put together recommendations for the next year's assembly.

I took this job seriously and worked very hard at it. I was shocked to run into the severe patriarchal remnants of the past that still held sway in this denomination. Women belonged in the kitchen or having babies, preferably both, certainly not in any governing aspect of the church. When I made appointments for my meetings I said that my first name was Chris, so they would be expecting a man. I took delight in seeing the look on their faces when I—a woman wearing blue jeans and dangling earrings—walked in to chair the meeting. More than a couple men got red-faced and a few were initially rendered speechless!

In this role my alter Christine was in her element. Always the consummate CEO, she was organized and unflappable. If the meeting veered off in a different direction or the room got too heated, as was often the case, she took control and always had a plan to get things back on course.

My participation on the task force and on the church board brought my own internal Board of Directors into contact with issues and practices that they felt were ethically wrong and certainly not congruent with the Christian lifestyle. Once the church board planned how to talk an elderly woman who owned property adjacent to the church into accepting semi-annual or quarterly payments to purchase her lot. This way the church didn't have to come up with a big sum of money all at once and they were also not prepared to offer her the going rate of interest. I couldn't believe that kind of discussion would even be held; certainly no one disputed being good stewards of their money but I didn't think this kind of deal was acceptable.

Then there was the revelation of another sexual scandal in my local church: the associate pastor's wife was caught having an affair with a married man—a member of the church's inner circle. Unable to deny the accusations they confessed in front of the whole congregation and asked forgiveness from both the congregation and their spouses.

John, not being the forgiving type, flipped. "You're fucking kidding, right? They have to say they're sorry and that's it? Of course they're frigging sorry. Sorry they got caught!"

Every church board meeting found me at odds with the rest: me against five men. John would let nothing go by, not the slightest hint of the inappropriate. What they deemed as being "good stewards" of God's money, I questioned as borderline dishonest—or sometimes blatant fraud. I would hear John in my head constantly questioning everything they did, never accepting anything on its own merits. He refused to accept things simply because they had "always been done that way." He knew these wealthy, powerful men saw me as a threat to their "boy's club."

At the same time the task force was wrapping up and bringing its findings to the provincial assembly. One of the issues was whether to keep an existing Bible school open or not. My churches were unanimous in their vote to close it, and the same with a majority of the other board members' churches. Just before we were to present our findings, the chairman of this task force and another task force member, a very wealthy man who was from the area the Bible school was in, hustled me into a back room and told me that this issue should be tabled until next year so that further study could be done. After a year's worth of hard work and negotiation I found myself being asked to sell out, to misrepresent what my churches had told me.

John laughed, "Swell, just swell, is this enough for you?" All the other alters were aghast, with the exception of Sally who really did not care.

I looked at the men in shock. There was an incredible war going on in my head, I am not even sure who was saying what out loud. "What about the faith? Wasn't this about Jesus Christ?" That was Chris's question and she had Christine's strength to back her up. They had done this together.

Finally Christine said, "You change any of what we have found and I will personally go in front of this assembly and tell them exactly what my part in this is, and by the way, Jesus Christ is still the reason I am here. What is yours?"

The assembly continued and the decision to close the Bible school was made. At the closing banquet, the task force was applauded for its excellent work. What they didn't say was that this was the beginning of the end for me. One man approached me in the buffet line. As he reached out to shake my hand and introduce himself he said, "Well, young lady you certainly made a fool of yourself. Are you going to be smart enough to keep your mouth shut from now on?" I felt my face slowly flush, I am sure I was beet red. He turned quickly on his heels and walked away. I wanted to run away, fast and far.

Later in private the task force members met with me and I was told in no uncertain terms that I was an outsider. One after another, stern men in three-piece suits said this would be my last assembly. "You have no idea how this church is run," they said. Another went so far as to say, "You just don't belong here, you shouldn't have been here in the first place and do you have any idea what damage you have done?" I was persona non grata, and they made it very clear that I was not welcome back!

If I thought I would find approval at my home church, I was wrong about that, too. At the board meeting you could cut the tension with a knife. The strong, silent arm of the male-ruled church came down on me hard. Many who had once treated me as a daughter turned and walked the other way when they saw me. People I had once prayed with, turned their heads, crossed the street, or moved to another pew if I got too close, like they were going to catch a fatal disease from me. It was an old-fashioned shunning. I was no longer their shining convert; I had become a thorn in their side.

I resigned from the church board. The three-piece suits were right. It was my last assembly.

John wasn't surprised. He sent a letter to Dr. Jurgens expressing what he thought about Christians:

Dr. Jurgens:

Now the Christians show up and they offer her something that really is too good to be true. A new start, forgiveness, how could she refuse an offer like that? She could make amends. If she was good enough, long enough. You know for a moment in time I even bought into it, I thought these people were really different; they really did have something I had never witnessed before.

But I soon saw it coming and tried to warn her. Once more she was being fucked. One thing you can say about Christians: they can fuck you with style, boy you are getting a first class fuck when it's taking place in the name of Jesus.

—John

I was devastated, feeling totally lost and alone. The church had been my family, my salvation, for so long. I had been the special convert from the outside: warm hugs, dinner invitations, accolades and special praise. In turn, I had put my all into everything I did there. Now it all stopped—not with the loud slam of a door but a quiet blanket of coldness and distance. Spoken accusations would have been much easier to deal with because I would have been able to answer and defend myself. This treatment was insidious and cruel. I had officially been ostracized.

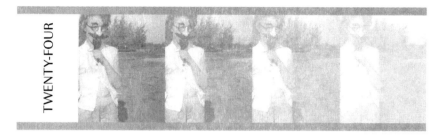

# TWENTY-FOUR

# *Revelation*

I arrived home one Sunday after church following the latest shunning episode confused and exhausted: a state I continued to find
myself in. As I sat on the edge of my bed, I thought about when I
had first become a Christian.

It was the first winter on the farm and I was passionately in love
with Jesus. I spent hours reading my Bible. I immersed myself in
the Word of God and the Christian lifestyle.

Once during that first winter I awoke in the wee hours of the
morning. My bedroom had been alive with the Northern Lights—
the aurora borealis. Despite the brutal cold, I put on my heavy coat
and went outside. It was so cold it almost took my breath away.
I watched the lights as they danced back and forth, their wispy
strands in every color of the rainbow, streaking through the trees
and touching the ground. I swore that I could hear them. Surely
this must be the music of angels, I remember thinking. It was so
real. First, ever so gently, they came closer to me. Then suddenly
they were no longer in front of me, or behind me, or around me.
They had encompassed me, enveloped me, engulfed me. I stood
still in awe of the wonder and oneness of being with God. Many
times I had heard people say, "You can't really know God until you

take that walk with Him." On that occasion I was sure God had blessed me with the knowledge that I was in his care. The lights were his message of eternal love to me.

But now, sitting on my bed in the warmth of my home I felt utterly alone. I tried to recapture that feeling, but it was gone. It felt like a story that had happened to someone else. Not even the Jesus part rang true anymore. What had happened to all of that? Why had my church family forsaken me? Why did God forsake me? Had all these years been wasted on a lie? Nothing I had ever been told my whole life had been true, not one single thing! The voices were strangely silent. The Board of Directors was quiet.

I was vaguely aware of a glass of water in one hand and the many pills in my other. Sometime later, I woke up to the phone ringing. It sounded like Elizabeth, "Wake up, wake up!" she yelled through the fog. Then I heard Rick yelling in the background.

I did wake up—in a hospital. I did not remember getting there. I'd had my stomach pumped and was not feeling very well. The last thing I remembered was talking on the phone and Rick being very angry. Apparently Elizabeth had called Dr. Jurgens and told him what had happened. Dr. Jurgens said, "Put Chris on the phone, now!" When I was on he said, "Chris, quick, summon all your strength, get to the staircase and call for Rick." Luckily Rick heard and drove me to the hospital just in time.

I blinked a few times and noticed that my mom was there. She knew I had been having problems with depression but had no idea about the reason behind it. I needed to tell her the truth—all of it. What would her reaction be? Would she believe me? There had been no love between Mom and Dad for years but this was something else entirely.

I told Mom of the abuse at the hands of my dad. After all these years that it had been bottled up, I just blurted it out. My thought was that if I didn't just say it I would never be able to. Rick was there, too. I could see their faces blanch and their mouths drop open. Rick really didn't say anything, which was not unusual for him when dealing with heavy, emotional situations. I did not mention the DID. I was still accepting that I had this condition so I wasn't ready to disclose it to my family just yet.

Mom didn't flinch or try to argue with me. She accepted without any reservation what I said to be true, saying, "I knew he was a pervert, but I never though he would do anything to children—his own daughter." At the time, I didn't have the heart to ask how it would have been possible not to notice what was going on with her little girl. It seemed like such a blow to her that I just didn't have the will to probe any deeper.

For the next four years, guilt and depression plagued my mother. She told me that she could not forgive herself for not seeing what had been happening to me, right under her nose and that she did not protect her little girl from being sexually molested for so long.

Mom had flourished after Dad died. She had finally blossomed and was doing things she had never done before. She had become an active member of the community, taking part in the local housing authority, the health board and many other activities. She participated in curling, golfing, slow pitch and bingo. She led a vibrant full life, finally not having to answer to anyone. She cherished her freedom. Now this came crashing down on her. She would say many times in the next four years how she felt like his evil could never be stopped. That he had reached out from the grave to continue to hurt them. Many times she would say she wished he were still alive so she could kill him. "Promise me," she would say, "that you won't bury me in the same graveyard. I don't want even my dead body to be anywhere near him."

While it was important for her to know the truth, I wished many times that I had never disclosed any of it to Mom, that I could have kept it to myself. The depression and guilt weighed so heavily on her that at one point she began to hallucinate, seeing Father in an oncoming car, and on still another occasion seeing other deceased people. My sisters and I begged her to get help, to talk to someone, but her response was always the same: "I'll never give in," she said, "they will just put me on pills." She had been on Valium once and it had taken her two years to get off it. She wasn't going to do that again.

The news of my father's incest impacted my three sisters in different ways. The one three years younger and the one fourteen years younger said they were sure nothing like that had ever happened to them. At that time they said they didn't know whether to believe this had actually happened to me or not, but they did support me and would stand by me, wishing me the best.

The remaining sister, who was ten years younger, had a very different, very dramatic reaction to the disclosure. She flatly refused to believe any of it and retaliated by sending me a hate-filled letter. She called me a pathological liar, and threatened me with all kinds of character assassination if I ever tried to tell anyone else these horrible things about our father.

I was hurt, but also strongly suspected that with the age difference this sister might also have been our father's victim. This was not something that I ever confirmed.

Meanwhile, the situation within the Board was something else entirely. I blamed myself for the state my mom and family were in, but not John. He was on another rampage. He saw no reason in the world why Mom wouldn't have known. Any time I felt bad about Mom, he listed his reasons relentlessly, fought his case like a professional lawyer and as much as the system protested and fought back there was always a shred of doubt.

"Why do you accept her explanation?" he yelled. "What about the throat infections? What about the vaginal infections? What about the blood stains on little Chris's clothing? What about the neighbor girl? What about . . . what about . . . what about?"

They were questions for which I had no answers. I believed her when she said she did not know. Surely my mother would have protected me. Would I know if my boys were being abused? I could not answer John definitively, but I know what I wanted to believe.

Despite my suicide attempt, relieving myself of the horrible burden about the abuse by telling my mother and husband was like a miracle drug. I spent ten days in the hospital and of course continued my therapy sessions upon my release. I bounced back quickly, overnight, in fact. I was delighted that I was still alive and that I would have another chance at life—now with my mom's support, which I needed more than ever.

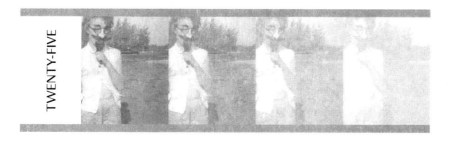

TWENTY-FIVE

## *Coming Clean*

My new lease on life didn't last long. Suddenly I started feeling out of control, as though everything was beginning to crumble. I was still going to church—hoping that somehow things would change—but certainly not welcome. I was a member of the Young Christian Woman's Club, which I helped form and had led from its inception, but even there I could not count on myself anymore. The whole sophisticated system of alters that had worked so well to protect the children in me was now constantly at odds with itself. Everyone seemed to have a separate agenda and all of them were trying to have their say—which was very confusing and often left me in embarrassing situations I couldn't explain.

For instance, once I asked to lead a simple twenty-minute devotional. I picked "gratitude" for a topic. This should have been a walk in the park and I had done dozens of these things in the past, many more complicated than this, in front of a much more intimidating crowd. Christine always did these kinds of presentations, always doing her homework first. She was never unprepared.

I was sitting waiting for my turn when I suddenly knew I was in trouble; Christine was nowhere to be found. I hadn't brought notes. Christine didn't need them, not for something like this. I begin to perspire, my heart was palpitating and I felt light-headed and weak. I was the little girl in the department store who had not learned how to tie her shoelaces. I felt like the ladies sitting around me were closing in. *Where is the Board? Where the hell is the Board?*

I started to panic and knew that my only option was to leave quickly. I tapped the arm of the lady seated next to me. "I am feeling ill, I won't be able to speak, please excuse me," I stammered, and nearly ran from the room.

Stumbling into the ladies bathroom I slumped onto the toilet. *What had happened?* I felt absolutely humiliated. *Where was Christine? In fact, where was Elizabeth?*

"Haven't you had enough of these fucking hypocrites?" a loud booming voice yelled. It was John. I cried, ran out the back door and got into my car.

These kinds of events began to happen more and more. I couldn't count on myself. That along with the shunning and the incredible guilt I carried caused me to withdraw more and more. *I am finished with church! I am finished with all community involvement!* I thought.

The only thing I really had left was my job but John continued to steal and the guilt from that was reaching mammoth proportions.

I had no idea what to do. Not only was I out of control, but my alters were out of control—and I was certainly no longer in charge of them.

Luckily, my impeccable work ethic had made me one of the most sought after workers in the area. I came highly recommended. Really, it was all due to Christine. She was a consummate professional, while I—Chris—was a homemaker. In many respects, Christine and Chris were at odds—the nurturing and forgiving caretaker versus the business executive who cuts no corners.

I was in a tenuous mental state after the suicide attempt and was close to reaching the breaking point again. I knew it was only a matter of time before John's embezzlement would be discovered. While he instigated and carried out every aspect of the theft, by now I knew him so well that there was almost a co-consciousness sort of relationship. There were times when I realized what was happening when it was happening, and I tried to fix things, to repair the damage he had caused. But now things were so far gone that some things were irreparable. I knew the banks would soon catch on to the erratic, unusual behavior in Mrs. McClaren's account, so it seemed inevitable this façade would come crashing down. Part of me was scared to death, while another part of me felt relieved that even if it did, that might bring an end to John's bullying and subversive behavior.

The chatter in my head was conspiring against John. "This stealing has to stop," said Elizabeth, over and over again. Occasionally she would add, "Maybe we can return it."

Christine would add, "Give it back, please, before it's all gone. Give it back, no one needs to know." Chris would just cry.

John smelled a conspiracy to be rid of him so, as usual, he became hostile and confrontational, "No one needs to know—get your head together! This is a sweet deal."

In spite of his demands the women made a decision to stop—with the exception of Sally, who really didn't care. Christine, Chris and Elizabeth displayed a rare strength and a unity of purpose.

I decided to tell my mother and Rick both about the theft and about the DID diagnosis. They went hand in glove, after all. "Rick I need to go to my mother's house, right now, and you need to come with me. There is something important I need to tell both of you together," I said.

"Okay," he said shrugging his shoulders. I cried non-stop on the ride over. He didn't ask why, maybe because he had seen me like this so many times before.

I walked through her front door with red, swollen eyes. "What's happening?" Mom asked. As I tried to pull myself together, taking deep breaths and wiping my face dry, Christine took over, immediately stopped the crying and launched into the story with her typical efficiency.

"When I was in the hospital, I told you about how Dad molested me," I said, wringing my hands, "but that was just the beginning. There's much more to my story." Then I told them everything. My diagnosis, how it manifests itself, the alters and their roles. Mom and Rick stood stock still. I carried on while I still had the momentum.

"It gets worse," I told them. "You know the job I have with Mrs. McClaren? Well, John does not like her—really has it in for Dr. McClaren, even though he is deceased—and has been stealing huge amounts of money from her. He isn't all bad, really. He just wants to shield me, all of me, from any further harm." As it came out of my own mouth the explanation sounded bogus, like so much bullshit—but maybe that was just Christine analyzing. It must have seemed crazy, surreal stuff to my mother and to Rick, though neither of them disputed anything, not one thing. This fact didn't cross my mind until much later, but they didn't seem shocked.

"The only way to make this right is to call your supervisor," said Mom. Of course she was right, but I was suddenly so exhausted I could barely think. Mom placed the call and my boss arrived a few minutes later. Mom and I retold the story—of an abused child who had formed multiple personalities to cope and how now that had ceased to be effective and in fact one of her alters had stolen a large amount of money from a client. My supervisor was incredible; kind, and understanding. She immediately put me on sick leave and on her way out the door suggested that getting a lawyer would be a good idea.

I expected Rick to be angry about this but he surprised me. He said he would support me 100 percent and would pay back all the money. "I had no idea this was happening," he said to my supervisor.

John was livid. "He is a not a complete fucking idiot; are you really going to let him get away with this?" he screamed. "Where exactly does that dumb fuck think the two-car garage came from and the fucking trip to Florida—from your crafting money? Right! Give me a total frigging break—now he's going to be Mr. Fucking Hero? Don't let him do this," John yelled.

I took my supervisor's advice and looked for a lawyer. The first one I approached just shook his head and said, "I'm sorry, I just can't handle this." I wondered how hard handling any of this would be, considering all I wanted to do was plead guilty and make things right. The only reason I wanted a lawyer was to explain the situation and keep myself out of jail. I had never intended to try and deny anything. Luckily I found someone to represent me. He contacted the Royal Canadian Mounted Police (RCMP) and they formally pressed charges.

My attorney set up a meeting with the RCMP officer in charge of my case. I asked Rick if he would come with me. "I'm sorry, I can't come. I have to work," he said. My stomach dropped. "You know, I have to pay off the $10,000 you stole so I think it is better for me to show up to my job than to go to court."

John jumped right on that, "What part of standing by you 100 percent would this be you dumb fuck?"

My lawyer decided the best course of action was straightforward honesty. I had a letter from my psychologist confirming the dissociative identity disorder. I had the erratic deposit/withdraw/deposit evidence to back that up, and I was pleading guilty. I was also offering complete restitution and had no previous record of any kind.

The meeting with the police officer was short and to the point. My lawyer advised, "Don't offer any extra information than is necessary. The young policeman had a lot of questions about dissociative identity disorder and it was obvious he would have liked to have asked more.

The court appearance was mercifully short. I guess I had hoped Rick might show up to support me after all but he did not. The court ordered three years' probation and restitution. I breathed a sigh of relief, feeling the weight of the world was off my shoulders, for now at least.

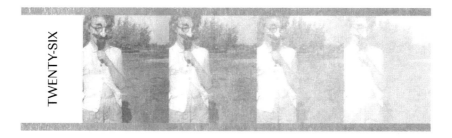

# TWENTY-SIX

# Up in Flames

I was in a neighboring town, Merrimore, at the open air farmer's market when I noticed a police cruiser paying special attention to my truck. He had driven by it very slowly, stopped and took note of the license plate number, then circled around and parked behind it. He got out and walked toward the market area.

I met him on the sidewalk. "Hello officer, I saw you looking at my truck. Is there something I can help you with?" I asked.

"Are you Christine Ducommun? Do you live in Riverdale?" he asked me.

"Yes, that's me and I live in Riverdale. What's wrong—is my family okay?" I asked suddenly worried something had happened to one of my boys.

"Yes," he answered, "Your family is fine, but I think your house is on fire," he had replied.

"You *think*, my house is on fire? You better *know* my house is on fire!" Christine shot back at him.

"I'm sorry," he replied. "Your house *is* on fire and you have a friend on the way here now. I have been asked to find you. Your friend will meet you at the station and will accompany you back to Riverdale."

"Complete idiots! I think your house is on fire!" John wanted to laugh in this guy's face. "Are all cops idiots? Yep! That's good, that's real good! I THINK YOUR HOUSE IS ON FIRE!"

"Are you okay to drive to the station, Christine?" the policeman continued.

"Yes, I am fine," Christine answered. This was going to have to be Christine's show—Chris was not up for this one.

A couple of people I knew from the church—the few that were still speaking to me—arrived at the police station to drive me to Riverdale and bring my truck home. *This woman must be doing her Christian duty*, I thought to myself. John retorted, "Won't she have a great little story to tell Sunday morning. Fucking hero!"

I could see the dark pillar of smoke from several miles away. "How bad is it?" I asked. "Is it gone?"

"I am not sure," the woman answered. "There were flames coming out of the roof when I left, that's all I know."

Chris popped up for a minute. "The kids will be in school, so they are okay. All my antiques, oh my God, all my antique furniture will be lost!" I started to cry. Nearly everything in the house from the master bedroom suite, to the dining room set, to the guest bedroom set was antique. All had what was called a waterfall pattern and all came with a special story. Some had been collected from my side of the family and some from Rick's. There was an old photo of my grandfather on my mom's side that I had restored and put in a special frame made by a dear friend, now deceased. Pictures, my journal, and photo albums I had spent hours putting together; so many things and so many memories. My mind was spinning.

Chris' guilt yelled inside: "This is my fault! I made us move to town! I couldn't live out there anymore! This is my fault! I should have been stronger! My fault! My fault!"

As we got closer to town you could see the flashing lights of the fire engines. The police had the highway closed off. There were cars parked all along the street on both sides and a huge crowd of people gathered. It was like a scene out of a movie.

It was a beautiful sunny June day. I thought, *Houses don't burn down on days like this. This isn't happening. They have made a mistake!*

"Right, leave it to you to think shit like that!" John made a brief appearance.

"Where are the boys?" I said to no one in particular. "Someone needs to call Rick."

I thought to myself, *I need to take codeine. Have I got codeine in my purse?* I was frantically checking for codeine, lorazepam—anything. "I need my pills. My God are my pills in the house?" *Am I saying this out loud?* "My antiques, this can't be happening!" I was shaking and crying and so scared that I *was* screaming all of this out loud.

Now out of the truck, we walked toward what was left of the house. Smoke was still coming out of the top. Mom walked toward me, crying. My friend Mary was there along with many policemen and, of course, the firemen. The front half of the house, where the master bedroom had been, was gone. The picture window was smashed out of the other half, exposing the living and dining room to the whole world. I saw the old antique phonograph cabinet I had gutted and redone, all my photo albums were in that cabinet.

Suddenly I yelled at the fire chief. "Get that out of there now! It has all my pictures!" I screamed and ran toward him. A policeman tried to hold me back. "You don't understand, that cabinet has all of my photo albums in it," I was hysterical. I felt like I was speaking a foreign language and that no one could understand me.

The fire chief heard me and, with the fire pretty much under control by now, he retrieved the old phonograph cabinet. It was soaking wet and covered with ashes. The albums were starting to soak up water but the pictures were saved. My neighbors began to remove them so that they wouldn't be completely ruined, and spread them out over the adjacent lawn to dry. My whole life, soaking wet, was out there for all to see.

A woman from the Salvation Army stuck a card in my hand and told me that anything I needed from their store in Merrimore was free for the taking.

My house was destroyed. People were looking right through the partially standing walls, shaking their heads. It was like they were looking right through the wreckage that had been my life.

I thought, *What will Rick do? He is too weak to handle this! He will drink! Where are the boys?*

Finally, I saw Craig and Cory surrounded by their friends. *God, how can you take everything from them like this? This just isn't fair!* I started to cry as they got closer. *No! No! I have to be strong! No, I can't do this!* The crying stopped as I walked toward the boys.

I shivered and felt my head tilt, then Christine took over. This was a good thing; the children needed strength and composure, not weakness and blubbering. "Are you guys okay?" Christine said as she hugged them both. "We are going to be all right. The main thing is *we* are okay. This was just stuff, guys; we can get more stuff but we can't replace each other."

Pulling out her credit card she said, "You're going to need some clothes right away. Go downtown and get something really nice to tide you over until we can get to the city. This will give you something to do for now."

"Did anyone get hold of Dad?" Craig asked.

"No. He must be out of cell phone range but I will keep trying," Christine answered.

Eventually she did make contact with Rick. "The house has burned and we have lost everything," she said matter-of-factly. He began to weep on the phone. She consoled him, as she had the boys, telling him the same thing she had them, only she felt nothing for him; she only knew she had to keep him together for the sake of the boys. She just hoped she could keep John quiet. Things were much easier when he was under control.

Mom said we could stay with her, but I knew that was just a short-term solution to our homelessness. Cory's behavioral issues didn't mix well with my mother's short fuse. Mom's nerves had been frayed ever since the disclosure about the incest, and she definitely needed her space—besides which anyone would find it hard to adjust to a family of four moving in with them after having been alone for so long. We needed to make alternate arrangements—and fast.

Christine hopped on everything with her typical efficiency. She handled all the insurance claims paperwork with ease and people marveled at her composure after such a life-altering crisis. She discovered from the insurance investigator that the cause of the fire was an electrical problem, not a surprise as the house was very old. She and Rick decided to build a new home on the same location using the existing basement. She hired a local contractor who assured them they would be in their new home in four months, at the beginning of October. It would be a fresh start and they could have the house of their dreams.

Where would we live in the meantime? Rick was working out of town during the week and was only home on weekends. Craig would be at camp for part of the summer. We all came to a rather strange but innovative idea: since it was summer and the weather was nice, we would become campers for a few months. We each had a camper of our own and joined them together with a huge awning. The middle area served as a living area, complete with TV, telephone and all the amenities of home. We parked all of this in a very nice municipally owned campground that had shower and bathroom facilities. For the most part it would be Cory and me on our own anyway. When Craig came back from camp at the end of summer, we borrowed another camper and parked it alongside the others for his bedroom. The weather cooperated and we had one of the nicest summers on record.

Rick and I got along remarkably well. His weekends at home were spent discussing all the details of the new house. He seemed to be very supportive of the things I was doing and had shown some gratitude to me for looking after things in his absence. He was happier than he had been in a long while. Our contractor was right on target and we were set to move into our new home on October 16—just a few weeks over his projected deadline.

Then one weekend Rick came home from work with an arrangement of roses, the most beautiful bouquet I had ever seen. "Thanks for everything you've done, Chris," he said. "We'd be living on the street if it wasn't for you. Let's celebrate and go to dinner."

John saw this as a big red flag and went into a rant: "When was the last time he brought you flowers? When was the last time he was this happy? Are you buying this again?"

Going to put the flowers in some water I said, "Not now, please back off, I can't do this now." I started to cry.

"Leave her alone! We will handle this." Christine warned.

"HE IS SCREWING AROUND ON YOU AGAIN! DON'T YOU SEE WHAT IS HAPPENING HERE?" John yelled.

"NOT NOW, WE WILL HANDLE THIS!" Christine shouted back.

The argument was exhausting. I longed for silence and sleep—and the only way to achieve that was with pills. We went out for supper and made plans to go to Merrimore the next day to shop for furniture. Before I crawled into bed I took twenty Tylenol with codeine. This might have sent someone else straight to the hospital but I had been taking them for so long I needed a stronger and stronger dose to achieve the mellow, warm state I longed for. I vaguely remember thanking Rick for the flowers and the supper as I slipped into a nice warm haze. For a moment all of the voices were quiet.

The day the trucks rolled up to our house with the last of our new furniture meant that we could finally move in. The stress of the fire had been compounding for months. Cory and I had lived in campers from June until nearly the middle of October, and Craig since the beginning of September. The novelty of camping had worn off long before that. Rick had taken off a couple weeks from work to help with the house so we could move in faster but this made for very cramped living quarters. I took more and more medication but found myself near tears more often and with no place to hide. John harangued me about Rick constantly, convinced that he was cheating on me again.

I knew I had to keep the voices quiet. I was so afraid of rattling John. I had in fact deliberately cancelled sessions with Dr. Jurgens hoping that would keep things quieter. When things between the alters became overwhelming, I would use a break from therapy to give them a recess. Psychoanalysis seemed to stir them up. I hadn't seen Dr. Jurgens in over two months, but now I thought I had better get in because I was definitely losing the ability to cope. I hadn't planned on it being the same day as the furniture delivery.

The kitchen appliances had all come earlier, along with the kitchen table and chairs. I had been so pleased with the selection. The kitchen cupboards were a rich golden oak. I had chosen all black appliances—fridge, stove, dishwasher, microwave—and even the kitchen table was black with chairs upholstered in a black, blue and grey fabric. It was a sharp, modern kitchen. The crowning glory was the sun porch right off the kitchen with its ornate cut-glass door. I was very pleased.

That day I awaited delivery of the living room and bedroom furniture, which would allow us to finally sleep in our new home. The boys' beds were being set up in their rooms and they were very excited.

My appointment with Dr. Jurgens was later in the afternoon so I didn't get home until nearly suppertime. It was dark and there was snow on the ground. Driving up to the house I saw that Mom's car was there. We hadn't been getting along recently. Mom was a very blunt, outspoken woman and she criticized nearly every decision I had made about the house. I tensed up knowing she was inside.

As I got out of the car, Cory called me from the restaurant across the street. Rick, Craig, Cory and Mom were just having supper, so I joined them. I really didn't want to be there; in fact I wanted to disappear.

They quickly filled me in on the latest. The boys had their rooms all set up, ready to move in, and guess what? Grandma and

Dad had already got the master bedroom set up, with the new bedding Grandma had bought, complete with matching curtains.

*Oh great! I don't get to pick my own bedroom curtains and bedspread! Was it something from a yard sale? Don't be an ungrateful brat!* A scream was building in the back of my throat. I choked it back. "We don't have the same taste. Why would you do this?"

"Oh, who cares? Thank her!"

"Thanks Mom," I said, trying to muster up some enthusiasm.

When we finished dinner, Mom said that she needed to get home. I breathed a sigh of relief. I walked into the house. The sectional, coffee table and end tables were still in their boxes. Then I walked into the master bedroom to find a very smart but very bold burgundy, green and white bedding ensemble with matching curtains. It was so masculine and way too bold for my tastes.

There was a fuss in my head. I couldn't make it out. Everyone was talking. Noise, noise, noise. I cried. I walked back out into the living room. "Rick, I am calling Dr. Clay, I need to go the hospital," I said. Dr. Clay was my local doctor. I had an arrangement with him that had been set up previously with Dr. Jurgens, that when times like this hit and I became overwhelmed I should call him.

I was so disappointed in myself and felt awful because I couldn't really explain to my family why I couldn't be happy about moving into a brand new house. Rick showed no sympathy. He rolled his eyes, shook his head, and mumbled, "Again," and something else that I couldn't make out and probably wouldn't want to hear anyway.

When I got to the hospital I settled into the bed and let the strong sleeping medication work its magic. I found myself drifting away and knew that I would have a couple hours of peace.

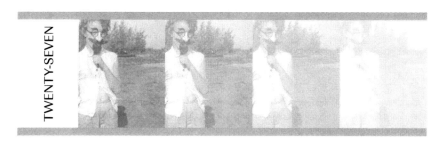

# TWENTY-SEVEN

# *Revisiting an "Old Friend"*

My world was getting smaller and smaller. I didn't go to church. I had withdrawn from the community. I wasn't working. So my behavior took a curious and dangerous new twist—or maybe it was really just an old twist. I began to drink. I don't even know why I started or where the idea came from. There hadn't been so much as a drop in the house for over eighteen years—and I hadn't missed it. I had embraced and loved the sober life; I loved that our children had grown up in a sober environment.

It happened innocently enough. I had been in Merrimore, the town I had been in when the house burned down. I was forty-five years old and had been seeing Dr. Jurgens for some time since Lynette had taken a leave from her profession.

I was grocery shopping and running some other small errands when I found myself parked in front of a liquor store. It had been over seventeen years since I had even tasted booze and I had never had a problem with that. During that time I never thought about alcohol, didn't miss it in the least. I went into the store and bought a small bottle of wine.

Later that evening, when I was confident that I wouldn't be bothered by anyone, I poured myself a glass. A warm, wonderful feeling washed over me and I had the best sleep I could remember in a long time. I hid the bottle, fearing my sons would find it. They had never seen alcohol in the house. It was several weeks before I bought another one. But I did.

❦

My therapy sessions were becoming more bizarre by the week as the core alters continually fought for recognition. It was as if they all wanted to talk at once and that it was the first time they felt they had a say, had someone who would listen, and not think they were totally insane. From the time I had told my mom, Rick and my supervisor about the DID and the criminal activity, there was an ever-increasing conflict, primarily between John and the others, especially Chris—me, the soft, maternal caretaker—and Christine. Sometimes it seemed John was afraid of the therapy, that it was a way of "killing" him off. Dr. Jurgens was afraid of driving John underground: without him present—anger or not—there wouldn't be the opportunity to heal him.

The only one who really seemed to understand that none of this was a threat was Elizabeth. It was through Elizabeth, who found her own unique way to help, that more and more was understood about the alter personalities. She often warned Dr. Jurgens if any of them weren't completely honest or might be a threat. More specifically, her knowledge of them and their importance and contribution to the system as a whole helped validate them and helped Dr. Jurgens formulate how to heal all of us.

Both sides of my family had a predisposition to being overweight and I had gained a tremendous amount during the therapy process, now tipping the scales at an all-time high of 335 pounds. This burdensome weight had become a major issue with me. I hated it. I was burying myself in fat. To compound this problem Rick was constantly whining about never getting enough sex. I didn't know how he could even think of having sex with someone as big as I was. After trying every diet I could think of, I became desperate, once again feeling like I was a total failure. I pushed my family doctor for a stomach-stapling procedure. Maybe because I was now morbidly obese and a major risk of being a heart-attack or stroke victim, it didn't take long before I was put on a waiting list for the surgery.

This was once again another desperate measure to fix everything, to make life better. I would still occasionally go into such a strong state of denial that I would absolutely, positively, convince myself that I would have the perfect marriage, the perfect life if I just managed things properly. During these times I painted my spouse as a completely wonderful, supportive husband and father. I would go to any lengths to portray the perfect family.

I—Chris—exhibited a lot of power with the Board during these times and could maintain it as long as Rick behaved, and sometimes even when he didn't. I was determined to protect my sons from the knowledge that their perfect Christian family was vanishing. I made sure the house was clean as a whistle, and attended to every domestic detail from flower arrangements to chocolate chip cookies.

For the most part John was quiet but he was still sure it was only a matter of time before Rick would get caught being unfaithful. If John showed reasons—even valid ones—that Rick was cheating on me, I just dug in deeper to show that I had forgiven him and that he was above suspicion.

At one point my denial was so strong that I even let Rick off the hook for a suspicious venereal infection. "Oh, that's something anyone can get," I said to myself. It was pretty hard to deny since I had contracted this from him, would be on medication for two weeks, and would have to abstain from sex for three weeks after the treatment was finished. No matter what John said, I talked him down! I was going to stand by my man. I remained steadfast, willing to hide behind the skirts of denial.

Another issue coming down on me at the same time was the fact that I wasn't bringing in any money. I had always held some kind of job, brought money into the home some way. Now I was on the waiting list for surgery and couldn't look for a job plus, with my criminal record, who would hire me? I wondered how I could make some money. Luckily Christine kicked into gear: "Let's start a home business!"

"But what kind?" I asked, relying on her to provide the answer. She did, of course. I had been a regular client of a reflexologist/massage therapist in the community for years, and loved the treatments, completely believing in the philosophy behind reflexology. In our family, I was the go-to person for back and foot rubs. This seemed like a natural calling. Why not, what did I have to lose?

Christine went into action, and before I knew it she had registered me for the classes. Four months later, she had studied and passed the tests for my certificate. She got me loans from the Regional Economic Development Coordinator which allowed me to purchase equipment and supplies. She ordered business cards, set up an advertising campaign, and painted and decorated the second bedroom in our new home. Soon Christine's Reflexology and Relaxation Massage had its first client. Christine's managerial skills combined with Chris' compassionate client care made for happy clientele and a good bottom line. I always feared, however, that if my clients knew about my past they would drop out of my appointment book like flies.

While the business took off quickly, my emotional progress stalled. The system was in a constant state of turmoil, arguing and chattering. Desperate to escape the mess of the noise in my head, I looked to a mixture of alcohol and pills for relief. In therapy everyone but John pretended that everything was fine, and John wasn't getting a lot of time with the therapist. In the evenings when I knew I could get away with it, I would get out my bottle and wait for the warm, wonderful feeling to engulf me and sweep away all my fear. If I had a hangover in the morning, I would tell my clients calling for a morning reflexology appointment that I was booked until the afternoon. Somehow I kept it together during the day—probably because of Christine the manager. But at night I would do anything to get to sleep quickly, to escape the horrible guilt from having stolen from people, along with the shame and overwhelming fear I had of actually going insane. I began to look forward each day to the fuzzy cloud that would come over me after that first couple of drinks, when finally there would be quiet in my brain and I could drift off into oblivion, up, up and away from them.

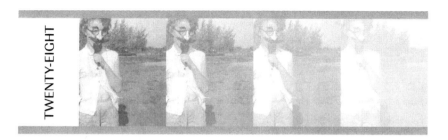

# TWENTY-EIGHT

# Betrayal

I was doing the laundry when the condom fell out of Rick's blue jeans. It hit the linoleum and lay there still and quiet at my feet, like a rock. Rick and I couldn't have children, so we had adopted ours. There had never been a need for condoms in our home. I stood and stared at it. Then I bent over, picked it up and held it in my hand. There was no emotion, just a strange overwhelming validation of everything John had known to be true. All the proof I needed was here in the palm of my hand, in this pathetic package dispensed for a dollar from some truck stop vending machine.

There was no storm, no ranting, no crying, not even a whisper; in fact an unearthly silence fell in my head.

In not much time, however, John was in complete control. Rick was driving his truck on some distant highway so John called him on his cell phone. In Chris's voice with Christine's composure he said, "I have one of your condoms in my hand. This marriage is over. You can be home in three days. That will give you time to figure out how we are going to end this." With that, John hung up.

Then he was gone. Weeping, I put in a call to Dr. Jurgens. "Chris, take a deep breath," he said in almost a whisper. "Calm down. We have our appointment scheduled at the end of the week and we can talk all this out then. In the meantime, promise me that you will talk to someone, to a friend, to ask for help."

I did. I went to my dear friend Mary, one of two close women friends left from the church who had stuck beside me without judgment. I spent the afternoon with her and even though I was in control, I knew John was right. I knew that in order to survive, in order to hang on to any remaining thread of self-respect, I was going to have to get out of this marriage. I could not tolerate any more abuse at the hands of this man, any man, anybody. It really was time to stop being a victim.

I had been so good at making it look like it was my problem that no one knew how horrible the marriage had been or for how long. I had worked so diligently at portraying the wonderful Christian home, indeed wanted my husband to be that perfect Christian husband and father, that I had convinced myself of my own fairytale at times.

Many, many times over the years in therapy I would tell of my supportive, loving husband, while the alters would be screaming in my head that he was anything but these things. Rick rode the coattails of my charismatic reputation in the church. He tagged along to Bible studies, Sunday school, and other events but never had any kind of spiritual leadership presence at home. Many times I pleaded with him to lead in that, but it would fall on deaf ears. I had begged him so many times to just talk to me—and now this. John was right. It was proof positive Rick didn't love or honor me.

This had to be the last infidelity. Three days later Rick arrived home, once again full of promises, the same promises as before. "It will never happen again," he swore. I had heard it all before. "Please don't leave, please!" he said tearfully.

I merely said, "No."

The next weeks were filled with arguments, both between Rick and me and between me and the Board. John was furious, "You should have had all his shit waiting on the lawn when he came home!" Once again he had been overruled. They just weren't strong enough to take the next step, which would mean living on my own—for the first time ever, completely on my own.

Rick tried to shift the blame on me, that I was the cause for his infidelity. He went into a long tirade about how I had never been there to meet his sexual needs, how I had been selfish and had made him feel like a loser, he then continued to say these other women had made him feel like a man. In the past I might have crumbled but it was not going to work this time. John waged a full-scale assault: "The low life, no good, piece of shit. Get rid of him, he will never change." Outwardly I held my tongue and let Rick rant, tuning him out like a bad song on the radio.

In the middle of this turmoil I got the call for my stomach-stapling surgery. Rick drove me to the hospital and was prepared to stay. "Go home," I said coldly. "Don't come back until I need a ride home." I hated him. I couldn't even think straight I hated him so much.

I recovered from the surgery nicely and the weight loss began immediately and rapidly. Everything was changing again. The reflexology business was really taking off. John was planning our exit from the marriage, and Rick was still on a campaign to keep me.

I sat each of the boys down individually and told them we were going to separate. "Craig," I started, "I am so sorry but I am leaving your dad. He has been unfaithful to me and not just once. I am so sorry. I know this is going to be hard on you boys but I can't stay. I love you and that will never change; I am your mom and that will never change either." As much as I tried to be genuine and reassuring, it somehow felt cold, voicing these clichés that everyone uses in situations like this. I couldn't really tell by the look on his face what he was feeling. He asked a lot of questions and said he understood Scripture to say that adultery was a justification for ending a marriage. He was pretty stoic, and then he got up and went to his bedroom.

Cory's reaction wasn't much different except I could tell by the look on his face that he was angry. He went to his room also, slamming the door. I know that this reaction stemmed from not truly understanding this very adult problem.

Rick's answer to all this was pure anger. He was livid. Though I wished I could take my boys, I knew I had to get away for a while alone. Being under the same roof with Rick was toxic. I packed an overnight bag and went to a relative's house for the weekend. It was surreal, I knew my husband could never be faithful; there would never be any point in trying again.

⸙

The idea of ridding myself of Rick was empowering but the reality of it was anything but victorious. As much as I wanted to leave him I did not want to hurt our kids or have to leave our home. We had been living in the new house for three years. It was such a beautiful place and I had a hand in designing every inch of it—with the exception of the bedspread and curtains that my mother chose, and which I had never bothered to change. I was especially proud of how I had managed to incorporate a screened-in sunroom off of the kitchen. It was a quaint Victorian style room; white lattice trimmed with green ivy and delicate yellow daisies framed the room and made it feel like spring even in the dead of winter. Someone had once told me that regardless of your color scheme you should have a touch of yellow in every room because it is cheerful.

I had made two bent willow chairs for this room and covered them with handmade patchwork quilts. A huge lilac tree was right outside and was awash in purple in the spring. I grew herbs and hung them on the wall to dry. I hung an abandoned wasp nest in one corner and an empty robin's nest in another. I loved this room. I could sit and watch the Northern Lights and not have mosquitoes pester me. I could smell the fresh air after a summer rainfall. Even when it got cold I would wrap up in a blanket and watch it snow. It was a dream.

I had poured my heart and soul into the place. When the house was brand new and people came to see it for the first time, I would show off the sunroom and say, "This is where we plan to sit and get old and senile together." While I realized this was just a fantasy I really wanted to believe that my life was as perfect as the house, as tranquil as the sunroom. I yearned for peace.

Ironically, whenever Rick and I had a fight, it was to the sunroom where we would go and tear each other apart. It was such a disconnect. He made the room miserable.

I came back from the weekend with my aunt and uncle, still firmly resolved to leave. Walking into the house with my overnight bag I didn't even have time to set it down when Rick asked me to join him in the sunroom. He immediately began to cry, he looked like he hadn't slept in a week. "Please, Chris, please give me another chance," he begged pitifully. Before I knew what was happening I said I would.

Where was John? What had happened? Perhaps Rick really would change; perhaps it would be better, perhaps, perhaps, perhaps. But what happened to John? Where was he when I needed him? Why was he so quiet? In fact, all the Board members were silent. Apparently the need to maintain a united family was paramount.

Rick moved quickly, calling the boys in and announcing that we would be staying together. The kids were very happy. So that was that. Breaking up, as the song says, is very hard to do.

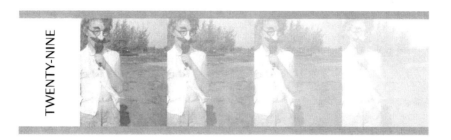

# TWENTY-NINE

# Sally's Story

Life after this decision was a mixed bag. My sessions with Dr. Jurgens had reverted to me pretending everything was fine. Christine concentrated on the reflexology business and made it very successful. With the new resolve to stay in the marriage, my relief at not facing life as a single mother masked any marital unhappiness. I focused on the boys who were growing up fast, and tried my best to help them navigate the teen years. I don't know exactly how much help I was, seeing that I was now becoming more and more dependent on pills and booze to get through the days. I was still drinking only at night, but the amount I needed had increased and right after the morning breakfast and off-to-school ritual, I was usually back in bed for a few hours.

All five Directors openly attended therapy sessions. Sometimes all of them would take a few minutes of the one-hour session to present their points of view to Dr. Jurgens, and that was becoming increasingly bizarre. I was aware of the strange confusion; I never knew what had been said or who had been in therapy. John was still hostile and vowed revenge. No one was safe and he viewed everyone as having a selfish, hidden agenda. His mission to end the marriage was far from over.

Someone who had been in the background before was now coming through more often and more emphatically: Sally. The drinking, the therapy, the weight loss, all seemed to set the stage for her emergence. While Christine wore a no-nonsense pair of pants, sensible shoes, a button-down shirt and small stud earrings to therapy, Sally was the polar opposite. When Sally was in control she would arrive in skin-tight jeans, a low-cut blouse, high heels, garish make-up and the biggest pair of gold hoop earrings that her lobes could handle.

"Hi Doug," she chirped as she giggled and sat down on his desk, crossing her legs and leaning way forward to give him a good view down her blouse. "Let's make this session a little more fun. Would you like that?"

Dr. Jurgens was a consummate professional who undoubtedly had seen and heard it all before. He responded in a no-nonsense voice, "You know we can't do that. It's not that it wouldn't be fun but it wouldn't be productive to you. Please tell me more about your relationship with the others: Chris, Christine, John and Elizabeth."

Squirming sensually she tried again with, "You worry too much. Come on, no one needs to know. It can be our little secret; I know how to keep secrets."

"Sally," Dr. Jurgens dead-panned, "Please get off my desk and have a chair or I will have to go get someone else to come and sit in on our session."

"You would do that?" she asked, her eyes as wide as saucers.

"Yes, most definitely," he said, getting up and heading to the door to his personal office.

"Okay, okay," Sally conceded, sliding off his desk and sitting down, pouting. This was her usual routine, and she would try a couple more times during the session before she really understood that Dr. Jurgens could not be seduced—though she never stopped thinking about it. She was a sensual being and was single-minded about the pleasures of sex. To her, there was no bad side. She never gave up on trying seduce Dr. Jurgens during therapy. It was what she did—and had done for many years with countless other men.

Slowly Sally's story came to be told, bit by bit, more often than not with Elizabeth's help. She would occasionally write short notes to Dr. Jurgens concerning Sally and deliver them to him. She would relate a deep empathy for her because Elizabeth understood Sally's purpose and her innocence. She began to recount some of Sally's story in detail to Dr. Jurgens until soon a new and important piece of the puzzle began to emerge.

Sally was eleven when her dad quit having sex with her. The child—now a preteen but still too young to understand all this— was devastated. She never understood why—there was not an incident that ended it per se, never an explanation. It just stopped. "What did I do wrong?" Sally would ask herself over and over. "I had always been his special girl, his good girl. He used to tell me that all the time."

It felt so good when they were together. He didn't hurt her, not like the man with the little Chrissy. That little girl didn't understand, not like she did. The abuse that had started out so painful and invasive had slowly evolved into something quite different. Sally felt special when she was with her dad and what had been horrible now changed as this felt good, very good. This didn't hurt and besides that he loved her. He had told her this was how it should feel. This would make her a wonderful wife someday. The other members of the Board, especially John, had tried to interfere but nothing could pull them apart. She refused to listen to them. They were just jealous, she would say, because she had her father's attention. That soon changed—dramatically—and it would devastate Sally.

Not only did her dad stop touching her but he stayed far away, sometimes he hardly looked at her. She didn't understand. She was sad, so sad and lonely, she couldn't talk to anyone. He had ingrained in her that what had happened must remain a secret, forever. Even if she could tell, whom would she tell? This must be her fault; she must have done something bad, very bad.

The same summer he quit touching her, he stopped going to

town with the rest of the family on Saturday nights. This had been a big family event for not just her family but for the whole town. Sally surmised that as her fault as well. Saturday nights had been so much fun. She loved to put on her prettiest dresses, the ones her dad liked the best. She had a pale blue one with a flared skirt and a soft white sweater that was one of his favorites. Lots of times people would come over to visit afterward. There would be music and laughter, and sometimes the adults would play cards. She remembered taking sips one time from the adult drinks until suddenly she was very dizzy and had to go to bed.

But her "lover" didn't come to town at all that summer. She tried to get his attention but he ignored her. It was like she didn't exist anymore. What she did not realize was this all started when she got her period, during her grade five year. While he bragged about what good workers his daughters were and how smart they were, he wouldn't touch her, like she was dirty or something. It seemed he was now sorry she was a girl, that he wished she were a boy.

She would make him desire her. By the time she was in grade seven, she'd taken her "I'll show him attitude" and ingratiated herself to nearly everyone. The goal was to excel at everything. She was always close to the top of her class academically and was well liked by her teachers and classmates—well, maybe that was Christine and Chris. She was athletic and played most sports well—a combination of John, Christine and Chris—very competitive in everything especially with the boys. Maybe she couldn't be a boy, but she could do anything they could do and better. She would make her dad proud and sorry he had cast her aside.

She soon developed a very sensuous figure. It was obvious the boys were no longer interested in competing with her on the basketball court. The first boy who ever asked her out and tried to have sex with her got exactly what he wanted and a few extras dad had taught her. Saying no was never an option. She became very popular with the boys but seldom had a steady boyfriend. Once in awhile someone would want her to go steady but that only lasted until they found out she was being intimate with someone else. Sally was just doing what she did, having a good time. Stopping the sex was never an option. There were many, many guys but none of them made her feel like her dad had.

For Sally it was just supposed to be fun. On a rare occasion, after she had been with one, two or more guys, she would come home and find herself crying. It didn't make her feel like she wanted it to feel. It didn't make her feel special, like with her dad. She didn't understand why. Sometimes this made her feel cheap, ugly, awful. Some of these guys were cruel in the things they said to her, or the names they'd call her. Her dad had never called her these names. She loved to party, to dance, and to be held close and kissed. She began to fantasize about becoming pregnant so she could have someone to love who would love her in return. She wouldn't find out until some years later that her father had robbed her of that as well because of the internal damage he had done to her when she was a little girl.

Sometimes she would hear the voices in her head telling her to stop, especially the angry one, he hated what she was doing, but they seemed so far away most of the time.

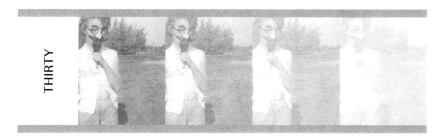

# THIRTY

# The Granary

Although John would seldom appear himself at sessions, he was now finding ways of letting my therapist know his thoughts on things, often simply by communicating them with Christine or sometimes Chris—seldom Chris because she was still very scared of him, but Christine was now becoming a regular go-between. Occasionally he would write letters to Dr. Jurgens, as Elizabeth did. As it turned out, these proved to very beneficial in helping Dr. Jurgens understand the alters' mentality and motivations. It was also helpful for me. I found this excerpt from one of John's letters especially insightful:

Dear Doug:

I was ten when it happened. Chris's mom was in the hospital having just had her third daughter. There was an old granary converted into a bunk shack for when they had hired men in combining season. By now Chris's father was having full-on intercourse with his daughter, a daily routine, as a matter a fact. Chris silently protested, and was always hopeful that someone would come along and rescue her—and us.

I told them they were all stupid for even thinking that way, because there was not a person in the world who was going to help us. And then one day, while he was doing it to her in the granary, we heard the door open and Grandma call out, "Anyone here?" There was a shift, Chris took over, caught us all by surprise. Finally someone would rescue us.

She stood in the doorway and watched her son fucking his ten-year-old daughter and she quietly closed the door and walked away. Chris began to kick and the others began to scream. It was chaos, we took him absolutely by surprise, there had been no resistance of any kind for years and this certainly caught him off guard. Oh, I was so happy that she'd finally fought back! We had the bastard on the floor before he knew what had happened! The victory was short but sweet nevertheless. Unfortunately, we got the worst beating of our lives that day and there was never any resistance after that on Chris's part. For me it had been worth it, but for the others it was the day all hope died.

Insight such as this helped piece together the various "noises" that I had identified years earlier, and it gave Dr. Jurgens a new way to approach a plan of action for our healing. At least he understood, as did I, that there was now a whole new relationship developing between the alters, all brought to the forefront because of the therapy process Dr. Jurgens was using. The alters were learning too; learning how to deliberately communicate with each other, rather than the previous operation that seemed to operate on its own system of actions and reactions to various stimuli. Not that there was anything predictable about it yet at this point, but there could be some definite communication initiated between them at different points.

The letter from John describing the incident with the grandmother also goes on to relate his version of Chris's life:

So what now, Doug? Now hope, now trust, now vulnerability? What has changed since our childhood? There is no more blood, no more ripping of flesh, no more trips to the doctor for infected throats and cunts, but what has really changed? What has really changed? We are still no more, no less, than a vessel created for people to fuck with, and when it's not the body it's the mind. Time and time again she lets it happen.

While I found John's words and assessment painful and his words harsh, I knew that his take on how I—Chris—had dealt with life was for the most part close to accurate. When I was a teenager, I was a pretty girl, and a good student, excellent grades, everybody liked me. My father had stopped molesting me, but what did I do? I jumped in the back seat with as many guys as wanted to be with me. After a few years of that and a bout of VD, I married the first asshole who asked me. After all, that is really all there is to life, just keep changing the sheets.

This letter was John's call to action; John was at wits end and couldn't take it anymore, and that meant that I shouldn't, either.

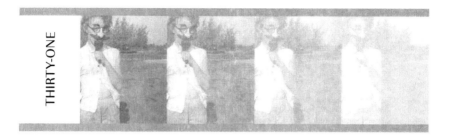

# THIRTY-ONE

# *Zoned Out*

While John got angrier by the minute, I simply zoned out, not knowing where or how to begin to change my situation. I was drinking
more and getting out less. While my reflexology business was as busy
as I wanted it to be, I found myself spending less time with my clients
and more time alone with the bottle. The more I did this, the less
capable I was of running it. My amnesic episodes were increasing
as well. At times I would have many things in my car that I had not
remembered buying: clothes, make-up and jewelry. There was other
strange stuff like potted plants, and groceries like lobster and huge
amounts of junk food. Whereas that had happened before when
the criminal activity was taking place and remained a daytime event,
now I was coming home in the evening not knowing where I had
been. I was never gone more than a day unless the boys were going
to be away at friends or youth club activities. I figured the blackouts
were because I had been drinking; I didn't suspect Sally. John was
still the prime suspect and after all why wouldn't he be? After the
theft he was the obvious choice. His retribution knew no bounds.

I was trying anything—pills, booze, prayer—but was sinking
deeper and deeper into depression. When I felt I couldn't cope and
that life was too overwhelming, Dr. Jurgens made an arrangement

with my family doctor to let me stay in the local hospital. This happened more frequently and before long every couple of months or so I would check myself in for a few days. They would give me a quiet room and I would sleep and rest. The rest of the time I hid away in my house, barely functioning, except when Sally decided to go partying. It was a bizarre rollercoaster.

Rick spent most of his time working; he also really wasn't interested in being around an emotional woman. Craig and Cory were busy with school, church activities, sports and friends. The kids were getting used to Mom being sick and having to go to the hospital—though they didn't know the real reason behind it. Rick knew everything but his way of dealing with all this was not to deal with it.

At one point Dr. Jurgens felt I should be admitted to the psychiatric ward in the city about 100 miles from my hometown. He felt I would receive better care; not just the meds and sleep my local hospital provided. While he was getting the paperwork together, John took over and bolted out the door of the otherwise unattended waiting room. No way was he going to be contained. Plus he didn't buy the hospitalization routine. In his mind, he didn't need to get well; he wanted to vent his frustration and anger—get even. Dr. Jurgens gave chase, but John got away and was gone for several hours. During that time I regained control and called the doctor, "Dr. Jurgens, it's Chris. I desperately want help. I just don't know if I am strong enough to hold John away until I can get to the hospital."

"Okay Chris," Go home and call me when you arrive," he advised. His main goal at this time was to keep us safe.

I never did get to the hospital with the psychiatric ward that day, but did find my way home—several hours later—and admitted myself into my local hospital instead. From that point on, Dr. Jurgens was very cautious about who was in control at the end of the sessions—hoping that I was—but it really made very little difference. In a matter of minutes after leaving, the situation could and often did change. There was really no way to predict what would happen and who would overpower me and exert control over me. The alters had their own way of surviving and that was changing almost on a daily basis; they were increasingly boisterous and ever more unpredictable. Rather than working as a system, now no one knew what was going to happen next. Everything was in a constant state of turmoil as each of the Directors fought for recognition and to take over the Board. As each felt threatened, each began to work for his or her own needs.

On one particular occasion Christine was in charge when I left Dr. Jurgens' office. However it was Sally who drove away in the fire red Chrysler Mystique—a peace offering from Rick after the declaration of separation. She stopped at the Boston Pizza Lounge and had a few drinks. She scanned the bar for good-looking men and when she found none she left. She continued to the liquor store and bought a bottle of vodka and some mixers. Then she hit the mall and went on a shopping spree. She had lost a considerable amount of weight by now, so some new clothes were in order. Lord only knew these "Mom clothes" Chris was wearing wouldn't do. Some new jeans, a couple of tops, sexy underwear, new make-up, hot earrings and several hundred dollars later she was on her way. She mixed herself a good stiff drink on the dashboard, put on her favorite music and hit the road.

Later that day Dr. Jurgens got a call from me, "Dr. Jurgens, help!" I screamed hysterically.

He said, "Take a deep breath, Chris, and tell me what is happening."

"I am at a filling station. I'm about halfway home from your office. I don't remember the session or even leaving home, now here I am, halfway home with a car full of stuff I didn't buy."

"Okay Chris," he continued calmly. "Are you able to drive? If you are, I need you to come back to my office."

"Okay," I agreed. But I didn't return. Instead, Sally got in the car and drove on to Merrimore, drinking all the way.

When she got to her destination she bought another bottle of vodka and decided that, after drinking most of it, she had better take the back roads the rest of the way home. However these roads were gravel, and driving too fast for both her condition and that of the roads, she rolled the car end for end several times. When I came to, I was standing in the dust looking at my demolished car. I was in shock and didn't really feel anything. I flagged down a farmer in a grain truck. He took me to the Merrimore Hospital. Sally and I had only made it five miles out of town.

At the hospital they put me on a stretcher, pinning me down in case there might be neck or spinal injuries. Luckily I only had a couple bruises on my abdomen, likely from the seat belt, and a bruise on my forehead, likely from the air bag. I gave the admitting nurses Rick's name and Dr. Jurgens' name. Meanwhile the voices in my head rumbled loudly, but I paid no attention and instead mumbled before falling asleep, "I hope they don't find out I was drinking."

I came to again with Rick shaking me awake. He leaned over and smelled my breath. None of medical staff had said anything about alcohol but my husband did not hesitate. "My God, you are drunk!" he said. He had a look of total disgust. He didn't say anything else and just walked out of the room.

This made John furious and he screamed, "The sanctimonious prick. Of all the times in all the years you have covered for him, made him look good, taken all the abuse, and he has the balls to even pretend he is above you now? Oh, his time is coming."

I remained in the hospital overnight for observation, and Rick came back the next day to drive me home. There was not an ounce of compassion. It was a long, silent drive except for John's voice. And it was in a different tone and tenor altogether. He seemed to be almost giving up, a different place for him to be. He actually admitted the only hope might be the therapy with Dr. Jurgens. Nothing else had done any good. While I found strength and comfort in his presence, Christine was impressed with "the big shot" doctor; Elizabeth was sending him notes ratting them out; and Sally, well Sally had the "hots" for him.

Whatever they all felt, I needed Dr. Jurgens more than ever. Along with my memory lapses, John had begun stealing again. He was using the reflexology business as his platform. Sometimes he stole cash, sometimes identification. He was setting things up to steal in a major way. Although he conceded that we needed to go to Dr. Jurgens, simultaneously something bad had kicked in again with him when I had decided to stay with my husband.

With John acting less outwardly irreverent and more in concert with Dr. Jurgens, my therapist began to focus our sessions on helping the alters show acceptance and value and worth in one another. In other words, he worked to show them how they could best serve their own needs, and mine, by understanding the role each played in my life, past and present.

Dr. Jurgens welcomed each of the personalities to the sessions and validated their importance, saying he wanted the chance to get to know them. Indeed at some of these sessions each of the five—Chris, Christine, John, Elizabeth and Sally—actually each spoke separately, however rare that was. It wasn't rare though for them all to be listening and to have Dr. Jurgens relay messages to them through whomever was presenting at the time. More times than not that was Christine's job.

Everyone, all the alters, liked and for the most part trusted Dr. Jurgens. They all liked that he wasn't a typical "therapist," that he wore his hair long sometimes in a ponytail; that he was a local boy from their own province and regardless of how crazy things got he never seemed to judge or look down at them. Dr. Jurgens was our salvation—but little did any of us know how long and rough the road to recovery would still be.

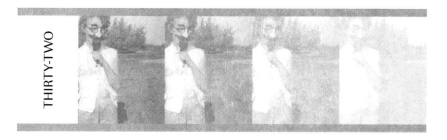

THIRTY-TWO

# *A Different Day, a Different City*

One day Sally arrived at therapy in her typical attire, but by the session's end, Christine was in control. Dr. Jurgens had a conversation with everyone who wanted to talk and convinced each of them that it would be best to let Christine be in control at least until they arrived safely at home. He spent a good deal of time talking to Sally and asking her not to do anything that would endanger the others; of course she promised she wouldn't do anything like that.

The next morning I awoke to find myself in a hotel room. The clock read 10:00 AM. *How did I get here?* I remembered nothing of the day before, the night before, even that morning, until I opened my eyes. The table tent on the nightstand read, "Roadside Inn, Kinley." This is a small city about a hundred miles from home. Apparently I hadn't spent the night alone because there were used condoms in the wastebasket and a partially eaten large pizza on the desk.

I got sick to my stomach for what seemed like forever. When there was nothing left, I heaved and wretched and then just cried. I was scared down to the bottom of my soul.

I picked up the phone. "Dr. Jurgens," I pleaded, "Please help me. This is bad, so bad."

"Okay, talk to me. Take a deep breath and talk to me," he said.

"I am in a hotel room in Kinley. I don't have a clue when I got here," I cried. "I didn't spend the night alone, this is wrong, all wrong. What is happening to me?"

"Is this Sally?"

"I can't do this Dr. Jurgens, I am so tired. No, this is *not* Sally." My body felt like a cement block. "I need to get home," I said.

"Can you drive?" Dr. Jurgens inquired.

"I think so," I replied.

"I think you should come into the hospital," he said.

"What for?" I asked.

"So we can help you," he said. "You need a rest."

"CORY," I yelled and suddenly became frantic again. "Where's Cory? He won't know where I am, I have to get home!" I hung up. I was in the car and half way home when I remembered Cory had spent the night at a friend's house and would have gone to school from there so he would not even have missed me. He wouldn't be home until lunchtime. I relaxed a little and once again I just began to feel very tired. Craig had been away at a youth event so I didn't need to worry about him.

When I got home I called Dr. Jurgens to tell him I was safe and that Cory was well. He asked if Sally was present but she was long gone, happy to have been out and to have had a good time. Chris was back and being a good mom but so tired. It was nearly lunchtime and she made Cory one of his favorites: tomato soup, and cucumber sandwiches.

After Cory went back to school I had a hot bath and went to bed, slipping beneath the sheets and into oblivion, hoping to erase everything, hoping against hope that I'd wake up to find this was all just a bad dream.

For the most part the Directors took very good care of the boys, often deliberately booking therapy sessions for Fridays and making arrangements to have Cory spend the weekend at a friend's house. They even made sure that those weekends coincided with times that Rick was away.

The reflexology business was a handy cover both for the drinking and the erratic behavior by the alters and to hear Christine tell it, it was even thriving. John snatched this opportunity to open up a whole new criminal enterprise: stealing people's identities and cash. It was in the days just prior to picture identification so it wasn't hard to walk into a bank away from home with a sob story about losing your debit or credit card and get a new one with relatively little identification, as long as you had a couple things with your full name and address. As relaxed and rejuvenated clients handed over their credit cards, John gleefully took a little "extra" to allow him to do just that. This supplied Sally with the funds she needed to party and go on major binges: food, booze, clothes. It was the high life, indeed. It was also a wonderful cover as far as never having to be accountable to anyone for money—especially Rick. And as for me—Chris—at this time I was so beaten down that I had next to no fight left.

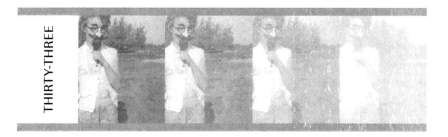

# THIRTY-THREE

# Another Day, Another Accident

The situations in which I found myself grew more dangerous and frightening. I drove down the road. It was dark and raining hard. The headlights glared off the pitch-black pavement, made worse every so often by the streetlights. The oncoming cars roared toward me, blinding me with their headlights.

There was so much noise in my head. *Where am I,* I thought. Suddenly, my car lurched sideways and I heard a loud scraping sound. I saw something in my side window, over my right shoulder. There was more noise. Someone yelled, "Stop!" There was no one else in the car. Frightened, I stepped on the gas and sped ahead. The windshield wipers beat against the windows like drums. I wanted to turn them off so I could think. The voices in my head were so *loud.* Why did they have to be so loud?

I looked in the rearview mirror. Someone was chasing me. Who would be chasing me? There were so many shadows. Who was chasing me? *Was that a car on the side of the road? Should I go back?*

"Go back? Are you a fucking idiot," John yelled. "You can't go back. Get off the street—now!"

With my heart ready to beat out of my chest, I decided this was good advice. John was the unexpected voice of reason. I let up on the accelerator and breathed a sigh of relief when I saw a sign for a Comfort Inn. I pulled into the driveway without hesitation and, after taking a few deep breaths to calm myself down, went inside.

"That will be $59.95," said the clerk.

It was a nice room, clean, tidy, and best of all, quiet. I was so tired. *What day is it?* The bedside clock said it was 2:00 AM. *Two o'clock! Okay but what day? What city? How long have I been gone this time?*

I rolled into a ball on the bed clutching a pillow to my chest and sobbed in desperation.

Then I heard another voice call to me, "Where is Cory?"

"Cory! I have to get home!" I nearly shouted, panicked.

"Okay, time to regroup, shit. Find out what day, come on, come on!" Christine was back.

It was early Sunday morning. I had been gone since Friday morning. Craig was away at a youth retreat and would be gone for another week. Cory was at a friend's for the weekend and would be home Monday. Rick will be home Sunday night. *That's tonight! Oh, shit. I have to get home!*

It was a quiet drive home. In the haze I recalled a lot of noise. *Was there an accident?* I'd need to check the car when we got home! I pulled into the fancy new two-car garage built with the stolen money.

"Right. BIG HERO!" John reminded me. "Hubby borrowed the money to pay the restitution and he played it like he had no idea what you had been up to. Interesting how you paid for a garage and a trip to Florida." On and on he reminded me of how Rick loved the spoils and now loved her guilt! I hated John's tirades, but he always spoke the truth.

*Accident? Was there an accident? That's right, I need to check.* I walked around the car and sure enough, although barely visible, there was a dent on the front bumper and some blue paint. I got a screwdriver and scraped the paint off.

I remembered the car lurching sideways, and recalled the shadow chasing me in the rain. *Did I hurt someone?* I shook and felt dizzy. It was six o'clock Sunday morning. I walked back into my house. I needed to have a bath. I needed sleep.

Standing in front of the mirror in the bathroom was a woman in tight black jeans and a bright pink T-shirt with the word "WHAT-EVER" in bold black letters blaring across her breasts. I looked at her and cried.

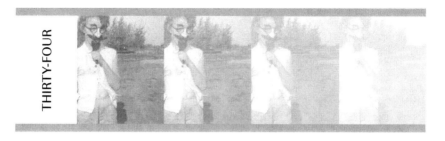

THIRTY-FOUR

# *Holding It Together for Craig*

Maybe one very big reason that I decided to stay with Rick after yet another betrayal was that Craig's high school graduation was not far off. I didn't need to ruin this special time in his life. John, however, was getting more impatient as the ceremony loomed closer. Rick wasn't treating me any better, in fact worse, and John pushed hard for me to leave as soon as the graduation was over. It was all out war in the boardroom like never before.

One day, with two weeks still left until the graduation, John was at his wit's end and rang up Dr. Jurgens with a new plan that would surely solve their problems. "I know how to handle this; she will never leave him so I have come up with another plan," he explained. "It will look like an accident, it won't be hard to do at all," said John.

"John, you *have* to tell me what is happening," Dr. Jurgens responded in a loud clear voice. There was no answer, only sobbing. He asked, "Is that you Chris?

"Yes, you have to stop him!" I was hysterical, "He has a gun and it's loaded!"

"John, John," said Dr. Jurgens in as calm and commanding a voice as possible, "If you don't talk to me NOW, I will call the police."

"Call the police! What the fuck? Whose side are you on?" he asked, incredulous. "There is no other way to stop this bastard, and she will *always* find an excuse to stay and keep taking his crap. You tell me if you have a better idea," he said glibly.

"John, this is not an option, you know that; besides if you did do this Chris would not be able to live with the guilt. She would be suicidal for sure. You do this, you WILL end up dead or in jail."

It was quiet on the phone. "John, are you still there?" asked Dr. Jurgens.

"I am, this is NUTS!" he answered. "It has to stop; she will never be strong enough to stop this bullshit we are living with."

"Yes, I believe she will, it's only a matter of time. You have to be patient. Now, John, promise me you're not going to do this or I will definitely call the police, I have to have your word."

"I promise, okay are you happy? I won't kill him—at least not today," he said, then hung up the phone.

Dr. Jurgens called right back. Chris answered in a very shaky voice, "Hello."

"What's happening?" asked Dr. Jurgens.

"He is gone," I said.

"Are you sure?" he said.

"Yes," I answered, exhausted.

"Are you okay, can you deal with this? Where is the gun?" he asked.

I answered, "The gun is right here on the bed."

"Can you unload it and put it away?" he asked.

"I can, yes I can," I said.

"Okay, please do that and call me right back," he instructed.

I sat on the edge of my bed in my beautiful new home, in the room decorated in green and burgundy, colors I hate, shaking and crying with the loaded 303 in my hand. The crisis was past. John was quiet. I unloaded the gun and put it away. I called Dr. Jurgens and told him everything was all right. "I have to go now," I said. "Rick will be home for lunch any minute."

Craig's graduation finally came, and Chris and Christine were once again at their best. Craig had wanted a big celebration with his family, his youth group, classmates and close friends. We put together a two-day event that brought all of those important people in his life together. This was an important time in Craig's life and I would make sure that nothing would ruin it for him. The behind the scene strain had gotten to Rick; he knew that our marriage was on life support and that the end would come sooner rather than later. He called my brother-in-law, my sister's husband into the bedroom to bemoan his unforgiving wife. "All I wanted was to make things right and keep our family together. She is determined to destroy us," he said as he started to cry. The crying quickly turned to heaving sobs, rendering my brother-in-law speechless.

My three sisters and I were in the living room just down the hall and we could hear him wailing. Fortunately the kids weren't around. We looked at each other in total disbelief. I was so angry at this selfish stunt of his that I left the house and went for a short walk. When I got back the crisis was over and everyone had calmed down.

John, however, was furious. "That self-centered son of a bitch! He couldn't even do this could he? Everything is about him! Not even for your son! It's all about him, about what he needs. He should have thought about that sooner; it's a little bit late to be sorry. We should soon be hearing about how she is the love of his life! And, oh yeah, how it's really her fault! Right! I should have shot the useless bastard!"

Luckily, neither this incident nor the subject of separation and divorce came up again, at least for the rest of the graduation weekend. Everyone seemed to settle down and focus on making this time a celebration of Craig, as was the way it should be.

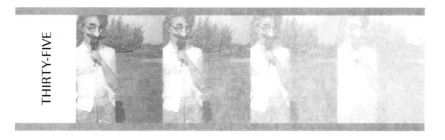

# THIRTY-FIVE

# *Losing Mother, Losing My Freedom*

My life took another bitter turn several months later, one cold winter day. Even though it is the natural order of things, we are really never ready to lose our mothers. In my tenuous state, I certainly wasn't ready to lose mine.

Mom was out doing one of the things she loved best, curling—a national pastime in Canada where teams of four players skillfully guide a polished granite stone down a sheet of ice toward a target. She enjoyed the precision of the game and also the camaraderie of being on a team and working together. She was a very social person and loved being around others and having fun— something Dad had really never allowed. When winter arrived and the curling season began, she would play at least once a week. She'd often join another three women to form a team and travel to weekend bonspiels (tournaments). When she wasn't doing that she would volunteer her time working at the concession area in the curling rink. She loved being there.

One day she was waiting for her turn, sitting on a bench in the play area, when suddenly she just fell over on to the ice. She told us later she never felt any pain, just a strange dizzy feeling and then nothing. She'd never had any heart problems before, so this was a complete surprise.

Mom was taken to three hospitals. First, she went to our small local one where they quickly determined they didn't have the facilities she needed, they then transferred her to a slightly bigger center about seventy-five miles away. There they kept her overnight and then sent her to the next biggest city another ninety miles away. Her condition was so tenuous that she could not even risk an air ambulance. It was determined she needed to be near some kind of medical center, thus all the "pit stops." At each stop, the medical team worked diligently to stabilize her until her final destination: a huge university hospital with a countrywide reputation for excellence.

Once Mom was stabilized the doctors performed an angioplasty, then placed a stint where they had opened a blockage in one of her veins. The surgery was a success and she was soon home and feeling very well. We all breathed a sigh of relief that she made it safely through this long ordeal, but our happiness was short-lived. Only a little over a month later, an unexpected clot formed around the stint and took Mom in her sleep.

She was only sixty-six years old. It just wasn't fair; not much about her life had ever been fair. I was awash in tremendous guilt, feeling that I had added to her stress during a time in her life when she deserved to be happy. I wished I had never told her about the abuse. It had shortened Mom's life; I knew that as sure as I knew anything. She had blossomed after Dad died. Out from under his thumb, she took on a new life, which had included getting involved in the community. Along with curling she also started golfing, and served on the housing authority and the hospital board. She was just a different person; happier than she had ever been.

After I had my first suicide attempt and revealed the incest, Mom was never the same. She couldn't seem to think about much else and became very angry, even if the subject of the abuse wasn't brought up she became very negative most of the time. I never forgot what she said, "It's like he will never quit hurting us; he has reached his hand out from the grave and it never stops. I knew he was a very sick man, but never imagined he would hurt you girls." It tore her up so bad, she wanted him back alive—so she could kill him herself. My sisters and I begged her to get help, to go for counseling but she never would. She should have been spared that misery. Chris especially wanted that moment back. It was the truth but what good had it done all those years later? Mom certainly could not go back in time and change anything. Instead, the regret and anger it had infused in Mom had robbed her of the best years of her life.

I had talked to Dr. Jurgens many times about all the guilt and regret I was feeling. He assured me I shouldn't blame myself for any of this, that the only person to blame for what had happened to my family was my dad. While I knew in my heart that what he said was true I don't know that I could ever shake the feeling that I had cast a dark shadow over my mother.

During the days leading up to my mother's funeral, Christine took charge and helped make the necessary arrangements. All the female alters loved Mom and were devastated by her loss. They did what they did best and functioned well during the crisis. John's feelings for Mom were more ambiguous, he neither loved nor hated her, as capable as he was of any of those emotions. He did often question the other Directors about whether or not they really believed Mom didn't suspect something about the abuse, but during this time of mourning he respected what was happening and remained quiet.

Craig delivered a short, poignant memorial at his grandma's graveside service that moved everyone in attendance. It was a bitter day out there on the cold, wind-swept prairie but he warmed our hearts. He and Mom had been close, teasing each other all the time. Oh, Grandma hadn't been real comfortable with his style of Christianity, but she was very proud of him. He was always trying to get her to quit smoking, always butting her cigarettes out when she wasn't looking. They had a special bond and I was glad, at least, that I had provided her with that much joy.

This year seemed like one disaster after another: dealing with the surgery, Rick's infidelity, the criminal charges. Craig's graduation was a joyous event—with the exception of Rick's antics—but that was a big change in my life. Now Mom's death, another very big and sad life change, was placing an incredible amount of stress on a very fragile system. The cohesive force we once had been was fractured as we all searched to establish our own identity. I still wanted to leave Rick but just didn't have the emotional strength to go through with it yet.

While Craig and Cory still did not know about my dissociative identity disorder diagnosis, the rest of my family did. The truth had been revealed when I opened up to Mom and Rick. My sisters and their families were informed not long after that and we had many discussions on the subject. I had given them permission to talk to Dr. Jurgens about it to help them understand. Two of my sisters did call him on more than one occasion and things that had perplexed them in the past suddenly starting to make some sense: the erratic, confusing behavior was obviously not the result of hormones or bad mood swings.

If they needed any more proof they got it two days after Mom's funeral. It was ten days until Christmas so my family decided to spend the season together since we were already brought together by Mom's unexpected death. Everyone was at my house when the doorbell rang. I hadn't heard it over the hubbub and conversation. My brother-in-law had answered the door and said to me, "There is a cop here and he wants to see you."

My legs felt like lead as I walked to the foyer. My heart raced, and my hands were clammy. This was unreal. *Not now,* I thought, *not right after I buried my mother, not here with all my family watching.* By the time I reached the door and took the three steps down to where the policeman stood, Christine was there. She was focused, calm and strong. True, I was guilty—or John was—but Christine and John would not show any signs of weakness to the man. Not today.

The RCMP was a short, stocky man. His uniform looked to be a size too small and his stomach pushed at the buttons of his coat. All the paraphernalia looped on his belt threatened to pull his trousers down. John sized all this up in an instant and smiled. *Crap,* thought Christine, *did the cop see that?* She decided he must have as he seemed to pull himself up as straight and as tall as he could.

Finally, he said the words I had been dreading, "Christine Ducommun, you are under arrest for a number of charges including theft. You will have to come with me." He offered this in a voice louder than what was necessary. The timing of this seemed no accident—they obviously wanted to catch me at a vulnerable moment. But if this officer thought that adding intimidation and humiliation was also going to somehow work to his advantage, he had another thing coming. He had no idea what or who he was dealing with.

By now my sisters and Rick had all arrived in the foyer. My brother-in-law kept Craig and Cory and the rest of the family and people who were visiting upstairs away from the hubbub. Everyone was very upset.

"What are you doing here?" Rick demanded, "Don't you know what this family has been through? Get the hell out of my house!" and he started walking menacingly toward the policeman.

Rick's unconditional defense of me and macho show of bravado toward the law was completely uncharacteristic—a fact that certainly did not slip past John. "What kind of fucking performance is this; a little acting job for the family?" John chided.

Calm and poised—John and Christine at their best—I assured Rick and the family they had nothing to worry about and I accompanied the officer to the police station.

The police officer questioned me for over two hours and tried every possible tactic he knew to get me to reveal more information. He got nothing but a smile and a request to call my lawyer. My lawyer told me to say nothing. I listened to another hour and a half of threats. Many times, the officer said, "We will come and search your house. We will turn it upside down and then I will get what I need. It would be much easier for you to just confess right now." But I knew he had nothing. I stayed silent. It was a crazy dance, a fight for power and control.

The whole scene was bizarre, almost surreal: a police officer and a well-dressed, middle-aged woman in this cold white room, devoid of anything other than two chairs, a desk and a phone. He could not, would not, make Chris crack—not today. The Directors knew it could wait. The family had enough to deal with without this.

I read the charges and a court date had been established. I signed a "Promise to Appear." Finally, looking the officer straight in the eye, John said, "If you have nothing further, you're welcome to search my house. Now I am going home. Would you mind calling someone to come pick me up? I am going home, this is over!" The police officer was fuming mad. His face was red with rage and the veins in his neck bulged out as he held it all in. He got up and opened the door for me, not saying a word. I got up and walked to the waiting room where my sister and brother-in-law had been waiting to drive me home. I remained totally poised and totally in control as I walked out with them.

"Arrogant bastard! What did he think he was doing?" John ranted, continuing, "Who did he think he was dealing with?"

Finally back at home, everyone was upset. I wondered what all the fuss was about. Someone said something to me about having explained the multiple personality thing to Craig, that he was asking questions and they thought it was time he understood what was happening. I nodded in agreement. "Yes, I suppose that makes sense," I said, and was relieved to find out it was one of my sisters who had delivered the news and not Rick, who surely would have laced the news with contempt and not compassion. We actually never talked about it, mother to son, but according to my sisters Craig finally had answers to why my behavior had been so strange and erratic for so long. Luckily, one of my sister's husbands had the foresight to distract Cory from what was happening by taking him out for a ride; he had no idea I had been arrested.

Another one of my brothers-in-law gave me a hug and said that up to now he had never been sure about this DID stuff, but now he was a believer. *Why was that?* I wondered. *We need to get things ready for Christmas,* I thought. Then someone said there was a call from my lawyer. *What was that all about? Was there going to be a search?* Someone said something about being glad Mom wasn't here to see all this—or was that in my head?

"Search," I said, "There's nothing to find, relax, let them search." Why was everyone in such a flap?

⋎

The winds of change were coming. Craig was in college now and would be leaving soon after the holidays were over. Rick was still trucking. Cory was still living at home and in high school. I was doing reflexology, when I wasn't drinking—which was starting to creep more and more into the day, along with pills. Now I had another court date to face—and possibly jail. I so wanted to leave Rick but now certainly was not a good time for this move. To say that John was unhappy about this was an understatement. I hung on for dear life and hoped that he would not destroy us.

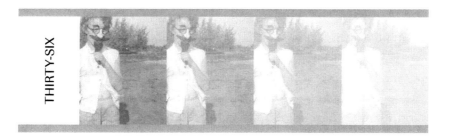

# THIRTY-SIX

# This Has to Stop!

It was inevitable that John's identity theft would catch up with me again. Living in a small town, and having a criminal record, made it easy for the police to identify what had happened when one of my clients had major bills coming in for purchases of liquor, women's clothing and groceries that he did not have any part in. A second major offense while I was still on probation for the last charges of fraud and theft could mean going to jail for a long time. I had intended to plead guilty and throw myself on the mercy of the court but my sisters, knowing the seriousness of the situation, insisted on hiring a lawyer to see me through this latest tangle. They knew that I needed a lawyer to find a way to keep me out of jail by presenting the pre-sentence report and speaking for me. They knew I could not do this alone. It never dawned on me that Rick would help, after all he was already being a hero about the restitution, for the money spent on him, that he never suspected.

I was overwhelmed that they would do this for me. The months that had passed since my Christmastime arrest had been traumatic and I had been in a very bad depression. The stress of the upcoming court appearance and the resulting conflict among the Directors had overwhelmed me and I had attempted another suicide in the early spring.

Rick had found me unconscious on the kitchen floor after I had taken a massive overdose of two types of medications combined with vodka. The doctors estimated that I had been unconscious at least eight hours when he found me. I remained unconscious for over thirty-six hours. Apparently the only thing that saved me from death or permanent brain damage was the fact that the two medications I had taken, though temporarily rendering me comatose and in danger of seizures, had counteracted each other.

My sisters rallied together and came to visit me, staying until I was out of the hospital. After my release, we all had lunch together in a family restaurant just before their return home. As we walked to the parking lot, they told me what they had done.

"Chris, we want to help you as much as we can. You can't represent yourself in court. This is serious business and you could go to jail this time. We've hired a lawyer for you," said Jan.

"How much is this going to cost?" I asked, somewhat panicked.

"It doesn't matter, we are splitting the cost." She added, "You don't owe anything. You need to focus on getting well." It was a done deal. I started to cry, and they all gathered around me and hugged me.

Tess said, "You have to stop doing this."

Between sobs my baby sister said, "We don't want you to go to jail."

We all cried and they told me they loved me. It was amazing and I felt so guilty for putting them all through this.

The day of my hearing dawned. It was a long time leading up to it and a long time while I was in the courtroom. You sit and wait with all the other people who have cases that day until your case is called while you watch the proceedings, presided over by the judge high in his pulpit. The surroundings are austere and the whole scene is pretty imposing.

The Board carried on a very animated dialogue as a couple hours passed before my case was heard. John's first observation was the noticeable difference in race of the people on our side of the fence. Other than the court officials, it didn't appear that there were many white people in attendance. "How could you have been this incredibly stupid?" he chided, "Look around you—the combined IQ here must be about 45. You didn't need to be here but no, you have to develop a fucking conscience." John was still angered because we had chosen to plead guilty; he was convinced the police didn't have enough evidence. It hadn't been too tough for them to put two and two together, though. Along with the male client who had strange merchandise charged in his name, another one of my clients reported a similar experience right after she'd had a treatment session with me. The rest of the alters couldn't deal with any more dishonesty and really wanted the stealing to stop so they decided the best way to do that was to accept responsibility.

There was a "hush" which came from Elizabeth

"I should say hush," added Christine. "The intelligence or lack thereof hardly seems to be our most important issue at this time, I suggest we concentrate on our predicament!"

"Oh, chill, you guys!" A giggle rose, almost out loud, as Sally made a brief appearance: "Sure would like to get under His Honor's robes—might help with the sentencing!"

The more time went by, the more fatigue set in and the more difficult it became to manage the Board. Christine and Chris were managing a joint effort although this was really Christine's show as Chris's guilt, remorse and fear were nearly overwhelming. What a different scenario from the one that had brought them there. What a hoot it had been! What a rush; what a rush for John that is.

It had been a blustery autumn day and John was in control. No one would know. Dressed in a heavy winter coat, a dark wool toque with matching scarf, and dark glasses, he was Chris, the housewife.

Striding up to the teller he had said, "I need a new bank card.

I left mine at home in my other wallet and I need to do some shopping today. Would it be possible to get another card?" She nodded and pointed him to the clerk.

She had said, "Certainly I can replace that ma'am. Of course, I'll need to see three pieces of ID."

No problem! He had a purse full of things people like to see: phone bills, water bills, driver's licenses—all stolen, of course. Combine these documents with the confused housewife act and clerks never suspect you of being a thief. It worked every time. With a new bank card and pin in hand, the alters were now off on another spending spree.

John was euphoric at their stupidity. He never had any intention of getting caught, much less taking responsibility for the fraud, so when the investigation revealed the physical description the bank employee had given of Chris, John was hysterical; he knew they couldn't prove anything. So why would they admit it? Why? He didn't understand this!

John was livid. There wasn't enough evidence without a confession. He had long since quit using the card and gotten rid of all the other evidence. There was no proof.

It wasn't that I hadn't enjoyed some of the benefits of the money. I wasn't a part of the theft, but I spent the money—on my sons, and John thought I hid behind that as a cover. So here I was, here we all were, back in front of a judge, "Damn it! At the very least we should have played the 'mentally ill card,'" John argued.

"Pipe down, John," said Christine. "This is serious." John fell silent.

The judge had taken a recess to read a pre-sentence report entered by my probation officer. I was still on probation for the first offense of fraud and theft. Catherine Jenkins, the probation officer, had put together a concise and detailed twelve-page report. It graphically described the sexual abuse and even mentioned Rick's infidelities. She also included a letter from Dr. Jurgens confirming the diagnosis of dissociative identity disorder. It read, in part:

Chris carries the diagnosis of dissociative identity disorder, more commonly known as multiple personality disorder, the result of severe, intrusive and prolonged sexual and physical abuse by her father. This abuse began when Chris was a young child and continued into her adolescence. As it happens in other victims of similar abuse, her personality split into a large number of "alters," a strategy which greatly assists the young and growing child in dealing with the intensely traumatic events which she is regularly experiencing. Although an effective and, indeed, efficient way to deal with this trauma in childhood, individuals who utilize this strategy very commonly experience significant behavior problems as they become adults. As you are aware, these problems have been a feature of Chris's adult life.

When I read the report, its words hit me like a boulder. Maybe it was because it was so thorough and right there in black and white for the entire world to see. Someone had actually believed me and enough so that they had put it down on paper and presented it to a judge.

The report ended with a recommendation to be as lenient as the law permitted.

When the perfunctory "All rise!" was commanded I felt numb. My hands were sweating. I felt sick. This was bad. I was afraid. I wanted to cry but I knew that I mustn't.

"HUSH!" said Elizabeth

"Do you understand that a period of incarceration would not be considered unreasonable for this offense, considering your previous offenses?" the judge asked.

"Yes I understand," Christine responded knowing that Chris would crumble. Her head was high, but not too high, showing just the proper amount of respect and looking straightforward.

"Have you anything you would like to add to what I have here?" he asked.

"No, your Honor," Christine responded, head still high. She remembered everything they had discussed with the lawyer. There would be little to gain by saying anything. The pre-sentence report had included her remorse and her intention to make restitution.

The judge leaned back in his chair and took a lengthy dramatic pause. Chris was near collapse and I showed it. "It's all right, we will be all right," Elizabeth had me in her arms.

John said smugly, "WE HAVE HIM! RELAX!"

"Yes," Christine agreed, "We are walking out of here!"

The judge leaned forward and cleared his throat. After slowly, deliberately, explaining the sentencing alternatives he had, he finally concluded that I—and the public—would be best served by a community based disposition, meaning NO JAIL! Instead he was going to place me on more probation. Of course, he added the condition that I must pay restitution and continue counseling with Dr. Jurgens.

"My decision to be so lenient is based very much on the reports given by Dr. Jurgens and the probation officer, who feel strongly that your mental health issues had been primary contributing factors. They both agreed that you have been making significant progress and are far less likely to reoffend in the future," said the judge. He added, in a no-nonsense tone, "Should you appear before this court again, there will be no such leniency. You will be incarcerated, have no doubt, do you understand?" he asked.

"Yes, your Honor, I understand," I quietly replied, my head nearly on my chest, my voice shaking.

Inside my head there was a party going on. There was so much noise I could barely hear his next words. They came from far away, from down a long tunnel. "You're dismissed," he said and nodded his head sternly but smiled at me and added, "Good luck."

I was so overwhelmed that I was unable to move. The reality of how close I had come to going to jail had hit me like a truck. My lawyer guided me by the arm out of the courtroom. I turned and shook his hand thanking him for his help. *This has to stop! We can't do this anymore! This has to stop!* a voice echoed in my head.

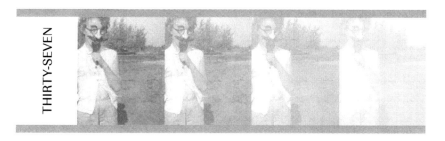

# THIRTY-SEVEN

# Rest Is Good

My freedom ensured, for now, I continued on with my therapy sessions. Five days later, the Directors and I sat in Dr. Jurgens office.

"I am glad you could come, John," Dr. Jurgens said. He could always note a change in my demeanor and thus who was in charge. John sat with legs spread wide, one arm slung across the back of the chair. "How are things going, for you?"

John shot back, "Let's skip the small talk. I came because I *had* to. You have to talk to Chris, to get through to her once and for all. She has to get out of living with this creep of a husband she's with; it's way past time!"

"Out of there—what do you mean?"

"She can't stay; it's crazy making. She keeps thinking he'll change but it's never going to happen. He treats her like shit and she takes it."

"What do you mean he treats her like shit?"

"She gets the cold shoulder from him. He's a waste of skin, never been good enough for her, never will be. She knows it; she's got to be half drunk to even stand being around him, and all the time he's playing the good guy to everybody. You've got to talk to her!"

"I can talk to her, but tell her how you feel."

"She knows how I feel but *she's not listening to me.*"

"It must be pretty frustrating trying to take care of her. Is that a hard job?"

"On some days it is damn near impossible."

"Does she know you're here?"

"Fuck no. She would freak!"

"I think she's stronger than you give her credit for. Should we try to talk with her right now?"

"God knows I've tried. If you can reach her, that would be great. Someone has got to talk some sense into her."

Suddenly Chris sat up straight, brought her arm off the back of the chair, crossed her legs, gave her head a little sideways shudder and blinked a couple of times as if someone had shined a flashlight in her eyes and she was trying to refocus.

"Hi," said Christine.

"Chris?" Dr. Jurgens asked.

"Christine, but Chris is with me," she said.

"Have you been here while I have been talking to John?" he asked.

"Yes," she answered.

"What about Chris, does she know what John and I have been talking about?"

"Well, maybe . . . but she's terrified of John, so there is only so much she will open herself to hear him. Can we talk about the court and what happened there?"

"Yes, but first I need to say hi to Chris and by the way, if John or Sally or Elizabeth is here as well I want to welcome you. We do have some important things to talk about. You *did* get lucky in court and thankfully you didn't get sent to jail, but that said, we need to work hard on making sure you don't repeat these behaviors. You have all worked too hard and come too far, and so now the work at hand is to communicate and pull together. I need to know how Chris is standing up under all this pressure. Christine do you think you can give me an accurate read on how as a team, the Board, as you call yourselves, is holding up?"

Dr. Jurgens watched as the person before him uncrossed her legs, folded her arms, put her head on her knees, and started to cry. Chris had joined the session. He handed me the crying pillow; I hugged it and cried.

"Oh, God, I am so tired," Chris moaned. "So tired. So tired. So tired."

"Yes," Dr. Jurgens said. It had only been a few days since the court, and not that long since I had been released from my last suicide attempt.

"We need to get you some rest," said Dr. Jurgens. "Is there any reason we can't admit you right now?"

"Can't. I'd have to make arrangements for Cory. I need clothes, there's stuff that needs to be taken care of at home," Chris said, stalling.

He pressed, "Isn't there someone you can get to do that for you, a friend?"

I shuddered and my head tilted—which I grew to know was when someone else was taking over. John raged in, "If she had a fucking husband worth his salt, he could do those things for her!"

I shuddered. "It's a very good idea for Chris to get some rest. Let her go do these things to prepare. I will be sure she gets back here," said Christine.

"I am sure you have the best of intentions Christine," said Dr. Jurgens, "but I am very hesitant to let you go. We have seen how these things have turned out before. You have all been through a hard time. I would like to admit Chris right away. It's the best plan. She needs it. And I need you all to agree with that."

Siding with Chris, Christine pressed for Chris's wishes, "I'll talk to John. I'll talk to Sally. I'll bring her back."

"Can't we do this arranging on the phone for Cory and for that matter even have someone bring some clothes in or send them on the bus? I really would like you to stay," Dr. Jurgens pleaded.

Shudder, tilt. "I am so tired. We can do this on the phone," I told him crying.

"Great," said Dr. Jurgens, "Who do we call?"

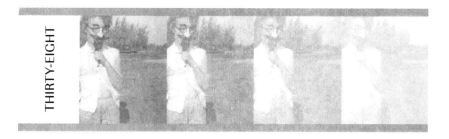

# THIRTY-EIGHT

# The Villas

The hospital called their inpatient psych wards The Villas. It was quite a misnomer: A villa conjured up a romantic setting in the south of France or warm sunny Italy; sandstone buildings with vine-covered trellises, a swarthy, handsome man and a bottle of red wine. It definitely was not this! Chris, Christine, Sally, John, Elizabeth all tried to wrap their brain around the whole "villa concept" as I walked with two nurses from admitting to this place called Kingsmear Villa.

First thing on the agenda was the scrutiny from yet another psychiatrist. I hated new psychiatrists and wished I could just have Dr. Jurgens admit me, but the way this hospital was set up only psychiatrists—MDs—could admit patients. Psychologists, like Dr. Jurgens, did not have that privilege. Dr. Jurgens promised he would come see me once I was admitted. I hoped my psychiatrist here was local—as in born in North America. It would all depend on who was on call when I was admitted.

There were five psychiatrists on staff and four were East Indian, so chances of my getting the fifth were slim. Truthfully, I was a tad prejudiced. When I was in grade ten I had an East Indian teacher who railed at length about all the ignorant Canadian people. That memory, along with the fact that I had a hard time understanding English spoken with an East Indian accent, left me painting them all with the same brush. This was unfair and judgmental but that was the way I felt.

I loved that Dr. Jurgens was not only Canadian-born but from my own province no less. I knew, too, that the dissociative identity disorder diagnosis was controversial—despite being written up in the *DSM-IV*, the bible of mental health diagnoses. Some doctors didn't buy it and that just added to my stress instead of relieving it. Still, I had learned how to use hospitalization up until this point for rest purposes—not really as anything more.

The fact that some of these doctors dismissed my diagnosis had messed me up for a while and I had even tried to convince myself sometimes that I didn't have it. Who in this world wants to be told they have multiple personalities? How weird is that? Certainly when I first heard the diagnosis, I was taken aback. The fact that some of these highly trained doctors didn't buy the diagnosis as a true disorder, well, that did leave room for me to be skeptical of just how much all doctors really knew.

The doctor—who, indeed, was East Indian—came in and began with his line of questioning. I didn't like him at all. Oh, well, I'd give him the standard routine.

"You are having some depression?" he asked.

Christine took over the conversation. "Yes," she answered, feeling the less said the better.

"Fuck, aren't they supposed to actually be trained in this stuff?" said John.

"How much depression?" the shrink asked. "You are thinking about suicide . . ."

*Was that a statement or a question?* I thought. I hated that this guy could not speak proper English. "I have been feeling overwhelmed," Christine answered. "I am afraid of where that might take me, so I suppose you could say I fear becoming suicidal."

"How things are at home? How much you have been drinking? What medications you are taking?"

Christine gave the necessary answers to get the admission. The subject of DID didn't come up. They were there for a rest and a couple sessions with Dr. Jurgens, so she would jump through the necessary hoops to facilitate that.

The next steps were about the medication and lying in my bed waiting for the beautiful haze to arrive. The meds brought peace with them; it didn't always shut everyone up but it usually brought some calm to the ongoing storm. And it did this time, too—but then suddenly something was wrong, drastically wrong. Twenty minutes into "the haze" my hands suddenly felt very warm, then my knees, elbows and all my joints. My face felt very hot as well. I looked in the mirror. I was beet red. I looked at my hands and they were the same color. Down to the nurses' station I went.

Apparently, according to the nurse, this psychiatrist liked a heavy regime of vitamins and minerals and some people, especially blondes, react to the niacin. Maybe they shouldn't have given me that on an empty stomach. The nurse said, "It will pass in about twenty or thirty minutes." I felt sick to my stomach, so the beautiful haze would just have to wait. Eventually it did pass—and I was on my way into oblivion.

Before I knew it someone was waking me for dinner. I was very groggy.

The dining room was nice with a high, open-beam ceiling. It had huge glass windows along two sides overlooking a farmer's green wheat field sloping down onto the mixed forest of pine, poplar and spruce. Maybe there was more to the "villa" thing than I gave them credit for. There was a deck off one side where the smokers went. I was so grateful I had quit.

I was slow getting to the dining room and was the last to pick up my tray. There was one woman, probably in her late twenties, restrained in a chair near the nurses' station. One older native man, who appeared to be in his sixties, was sleeping restrained in a bed in an open area. Probably detox, I thought. There was another middle-aged lady eating in a recliner. The rest of the patients were sitting at the dining tables. There was some conversation going on between a few people at one end of a table. It looked like they had been here awhile. The Board and I would get to know them, maybe, after I emerged from the haze a few days later.

❧

The rooms were small but private. I liked that they had pine ceilings. It was certainly better than the standard white tiles with the little holes. I had been in so many hospital beds and had stared up at so many white tile ceilings with holes. I would hopelessly try to count them to pass the time. I liked this ceiling. It felt different: peaceful and calm. What was it about wood that felt so warm and inviting? It made me think about my friend Mary. I thought back and tried to remember when Mary and I had met. It seemed that we had been friends forever.

We had that kind of interesting friendship that blossoms imme-diately and stays forever. Shortly after my baby daughter had died, when we had just moved to the outskirts of town, we built a large addition to the existing house that featured a tongue-and-groove pine ceiling like the one in my room now. Mary had begun to visit me there so that was why I thought of Mary now. We knew each other before that, but that was where the friendship had blos-somed and grown.

Mary had encouraged me to join a ladies' weekly Bible study and come to church. She had been instrumental in my becoming a Christian. We had shared so much together, so many laughs, so many dreams, so many tears. We had spent hours praying together for our families, friends and community. Regardless of what had gone on or how crazy things had become, she never judged me. I was thankful that she was a faithful friend, one of the few from the church who had stood beside me after I had been ostracized.

When I didn't have the church left anymore and the condom fell at my feet that fateful day—when all I felt was that my world

*Living with Multiple Personalities*

was falling apart—it was to Mary's door I fled and it was Mary who held me as I wept.

The condom had been the last straw for John. Even though some time had passed since that had happened he refused to let up; he wouldn't let me bury my head in the sand anymore. I had to look at my marriage for what it was—closer to a nightmare than a dream. John wouldn't let me hide anymore. The first few months had been fun, we had enjoyed setting up house together, the sex was good, and the parties were often, but when I became bored with the partying and wanted to settle down, a rift grew between us that only get worse over time. Even when the partying and drinking stopped there was not enough feeling between us for the marriage to be called good. In truth it was dead on arrival. And I had been the only one who had ever worked to make it survive.

I tried to remember exactly when my husband had quit caring, but all in all, I had to admit that maybe he never did. I could never patch together snippets of happiness into an overall portrait of contentment. I just needed to get it that my husband simply did not love me, and that a white-hot sex life in those early years didn't mean that I was loved at any point in time.

Rick couldn't even be responsible to be caring, really. I had a long laundry list of all the times when he had failed to show even a modicum of compassion. Like the terrible days of my hysterectomy. Where had he been for that? I had driven myself to the hospital, had surgery and then seven days later, had driven myself home because he was "too busy." I lied to hospital staff and said a friend was picking me up then I snuck out of the waiting room. He came once to visit but while at my bedside picked a fight. Instead of reassuring me that I would be okay, that as lovers we would be okay, he just fueled my sadness and despair.

Despite the fact that he couldn't be bothered to pick me up after the major surgery, he wanted sex from me the day I got home. This, of course, was completely against the doctor's orders of a six-week waiting period. It was always all about him, my feelings or health be damned.

I needed gall bladder surgery six months later that same year. Why wouldn't I be able to drive myself to and from that surgery since I had done it before? Hubby had asked. Those were the sober years, the Christian years, the best shot for a good marriage—they simply amplified how unsuited we were for each other.

So with the realization that there was indeed nothing left now I just felt sick over all the time I'd wasted. I reached for the pillow, rolled up in a ball, and cried myself to sleep.

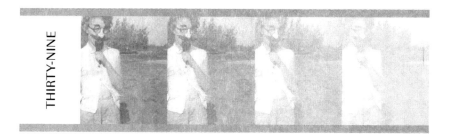

# THIRTY-NINE

# Attention: This Is a Looney Bin!

"Time for dinner Chris," the nurse said as she stuck her head in the door.

"I will be right there," Sally, answered, as she got out of bed and walked over to the mirror.

"Yuck," Sally said, "I'm going to have to do something about that!" She fumbled around in the bag her friend Janice had sent her until she found her make-up. Soon enough she had applied her mascara, some eye shadow, blush and some lipstick. *What's this? Great, Janice even sent me some earrings* she thought. They weren't her favorites but they would do, long dangling ones with purple hearts on the end. She ran a brush through her hair. *I will work on that when I have more time* she thought. She made a face as she looked at her blouse and then at the clothes in the closet. *So old, so frumpy.*

The nurse was back, "Are you coming Chris? You look nice, are you feeling better?"

"Sure am. Be right there!" Sally answered and followed the nurse down the hall.

She hoped no one was sitting beside Gary—he was good looking and she was sweet on him. Gary was in his early to mid forties.

He had gone grey prematurely—the handsome kind of grey, not a pure white or salt-and-pepper, but soft, even silver. Combine that with his light olive complexion, which was either a tan or perhaps his ethnic origin, and he turned heads. She wondered if he might be Greek or Italian, except he also had wonderful clear blue eyes. He wasn't a big man, probably five-foot-eight, very well built with square shoulders, a small waist, and a round firm bum that looked ever so nice in the stonewashed jeans he wore. Gary was quiet. She had seen him visiting with a couple of the other residents a few times but he never stayed around anyone long.

The big Indian had graduated from the bed in the dining room to a recliner against the wall. Sitting upright, Sally realized that he was not just big, but enormous. He had a tray of food in front of him. He didn't look very interested in eating. In fact he didn't look very interested in breathing.

Sally saw a chair open up right across from Gary and moved in. "What's in the little boxes today?" She asked as she put down her tray, giving Gary one of her best smiles.

The food was served in typical hospital style with everything in tidy little covered containers.

Gary smiled back. He had such a sweet smile. "I had lasagna today," he said, "and my soup was cream of mushroom. Some people had fried chicken."

By now the table was emptying and she hoped Gary would stay.

"Looks like lasagna for me, too," Sally said, smiling at him again. *I wonder what his story is,* she thought. *You look so normal. You look way better than normal.* She giggled.

He was starting to fidget, like he was getting ready to leave.

"Are you from here?" she asked. *Shit, stupid question, too personal; never ask a question like that, at least not right away.*

"I am now, but not always. I come from Toronto," he answered and he smiled again. *Phew, she had got away with it.*

"Toronto, wow, cool. I would love to visit there someday," she replied.

"No you wouldn't," he said, and picked up his tray and took it back to the kitchen.

She finished her dinner by herself.

*Brilliant,* a voice in her head chirped, or was it a thought? It was hard to tell the difference sometimes. Guess, it didn't matter a whole lot now, did it? What was a voice to one was a thought to another and vice-versa. *Keep that kind of thinking to yourself,* the voice said. Or was it a thought? *You get caught thinking out loud and the next thing you know you're going to end up in a looney bin talking to yourself. Oops was that out loud? Nope! Well, like that would stand out in a big way around here.* The voice again, or a thought. *Hilarious, fucking hilarious, end up in a looney bin.*

ATTENTION: THIS IS A LOONEY BIN!

Sally started humming a song from the popular folk music group, the Mamas and the Papas. She wondered if Gary liked to dance. Sally loved to dance. She took her dinner tray back to the kitchen and decided to see who was in the activity room. It was empty. There was a pretty jigsaw puzzle started on the table. It was of bright yellow poppies set against a rich blue mountain background. She remembered someone telling her that yellow was a happy color.

A shudder and a tilt and I, Chris, was back. I decided to settle in and work on the puzzle. There was a radio playing country music. I liked this style but felt like hearing old time rock and roll. I fidgeted with the dial and stopped when I found "Downtown" by Petula Clark. I smiled and started doing the puzzle.

The conversation in my head had quieted. It was a peaceful time, a restful time. I enjoyed the music and the puzzle. Yellow is a happy color.

There was a glass window in the door of the activity room that looked out to the nurses' station. I could see some of the smokers starting to pace back and forth by the door. It must be nearing the hour. I saw Gary walk past the window. He glanced in at me and smiled. I wished he would come in and talk to me.

After they had all been given their cigarettes I decided to join them out on the deck. It was a nice evening. There was a soft warm summer breeze coming in off the wheat field. There were smokers all puffing away. "You are all so inbred!" a woman in leather wrist restraints suddenly ranted. "There are no pure blood lines anymore!" She inhaled the last of her cigarette and stormed back inside. Gary walked in and I followed him.

"What are we watching?" Christine asked as she sat down beside Gary in the television room.

"*Law and Order*," he answered, "Do you like it? We can change it if you want to watch something else."

Shudder and tilt. "No, that's okay, doesn't matter to me," she smiled widely at him. Sally was back. *He is so handsome.*

"You're a very nice lady," he said smiling.

"Thank you," she giggled. "What a nice thing to say."

"And you're pretty, too," he said looking away, fidgeting in his chair.

"Gee, thanks," she giggled again. "You seem really nice too."

"I have been here a month," he paused for a second. "I am seeing my doctor tomorrow and will probably get to go home on the weekend; that's in two days."

She didn't know what to say. She was sad he would be going home so soon. There was something sad in his face.

Shudder and tilt. "You must be excited to be going home." Elizabeth had joined the conversation.

"Yes and no," he said and continued on, "Before I got sick this last time and had to come into the hospital I did some crazy stuff, so I have to live somewhere else now. I don't like that. I liked where I was living, but it will be good to get back to work," he answered, looking sad.

"Do you know what schizophrenia is?" he asked. He had now shifted positions in his chair so he could look directly at her.

"Yes, I know what it is," Elizabeth answered, "but I don't know a lot about it. Do you know what multiple personality disorder is?" Elizabeth asked the question but Chris, Christine, John and Sally all watched him closely, waiting for his answer.

A smile came across his face. He leaned back in his chair. Neither of them said a word. Everyone sat quietly. Then he turned to her. "Your voices are inside your head, my voices are outside mine. Mine are quiet now; they stay quiet if I take my medication. I quit taking my medication. I got sick and lots of crazy stuff happened. I scared my wife. She won't let me come home. I have to find a new place to live. Do yours tell you crazy things, make you do crazy things?" he asked. His blue eyes were full of sadness.

"It's sort of the same, I know I have done some crazy things," I answered.

"Because of them?" he asked.

"Yes," I said, not really knowing how to fully explain, "because of them."

"Don't try and blame this on me," I heard Sally say. "None of this is my fault, if you're trying to blame this on me, I'll come right out there and tell him myself. Why are you telling him this stuff?"

*Please Sally not now,* I thought.

"You're making us look crazy, stop it!" Sally pleaded. "He is starting to like us!"

Gary leaned back in his chair and sat quietly. Elizabeth and I took our cue from him and sat quietly, too. Sally was quiet. It was a nice quiet. There was no need to explain.

I knew they had started to cut back my medications because Sally had been presenting a fair amount, meaning that she had been the life of the party for the last couple days. She was first out in the morning helping to set the tables and she and the huge native, who had come through the delirium tremors associated with alcohol withdrawal, had even struck up a friendship.

What a character he had proven to be once he had quit puking his guts out and had a few good meals stay down. One day he walked into the activity room in the morning after breakfast where Chris and Sally were doing a jigsaw puzzle.

"What's your name, white woman?" he asked in a deep booming voice.

We looked back at him and said, "Chris. What's yours, brown man?"

They had both burst out laughing and were instant friends.

"I'm Jake and you are the whitest woman I have ever seen," he said.

To which we answered, "You should have seen yourself three days ago; you were damn near this white."

"Oh, that was a bad thing I did, I should have died, that was a rotten batch of homebrew I got into," he replied.

We laughed. "How many gallons of homebrew does it take to knock an Indian your size down?" we asked.

There were four or five other people in the activity room by this time and everyone was laughing so hard and making so much noise the nurses came to check and see what was going on. Jake was laughing so hard tears were running down his face. "White woman," he said looking at me, "if I didn't already have a wife I would have to marry you!" which sent the room into another fit of laughter.

Jake was a raging alcoholic, brilliant, with a charismatic personality and a cracker-jack wit. He was in his late sixties and loved to talk; and talk he and Chris, Christine, Sally and Elizabeth did. He hadn't started his drinking "career" until later in life. When he recognized he had a problem, he had a fifteen-year stretch of sobriety. Because of this the alcohol hadn't done the amount of damage you would expect of a man of his age.

Jake came from a reservation in the northern part of the province and, like many young Indians, had been grabbed up as a kid and spirited off to the Whiteman's Residential School. He had been fortunate in that he had escaped the sexual and physical abuse many had suffered, but he talked openly of being robbed of a culture and a way of life.

He liked to throw in a story once in awhile that had a ring of untruth to it, just to see if I was listening. When I would call him on it, he would throw his head back and we would both roar with laughter—to which he would usually say "You're still the whitest woman

I have ever met!" or "You're pretty smart for a white woman." Our exchanges were so entertaining they usually attracted an audience, but occasionally we would have some time together alone. That's when serious things, personal things, came into the conversation.

Out of the blue one day Jake asked, "What brings this pretty white lady with so much laughter here?" I instantly started crying. I had no words. He had completely blindsided me. With a shudder and a quick tilt of the head Christine shook the tears away.

He reached across the table with his huge brown hand. It was nearly twice the size of hers. He placed it softly on hers. It was so warm, so big, and so safe. She couldn't move. She sat and looked into his huge rugged brown face, into his deep brown almost black eyes.

"Someone has hurt this lady's spirit bad," he said and took his hand away. "You know white lady you cannot laugh away the pain, only tears can wash away the pain. It's soon time for you to let the tears wash away the pain."

"Oh what do you know? Now you're my shrink? I suppose you charge *really* white women double." Christine answered. It was a half-hearted, feeble attempt at humor, but this was way too uncomfortable.

Jake leaned back in his chair and placing his hands behind his head said, "Yep, damn straight I am going to marry you white woman. That's what you need. I will teach you how to make bannock, chew moose hide, and every night, after I come in from the hunt . . ." He stopped there.

We were both off in fits of laughter again. Jake hadn't lived like an Indian since he was a kid. He lived in a large city a few hundred miles away. The only hunting he did or had ever done was for homebrew or beer.

"I thought you were married," I choked out between laughs.

"Oh, my old lady won't mind, as long as you stay in the basement and bring beer," Jake said using the thickest native accent he could muster.

Maureen, the woman with the wrist restraints, entered the room in full rant again about pure blood lines. I thought this was a good time to leave the room.

Elizabeth asked, "Should I try and talk to her, what should I say? The poor girl."

*"WE DON'T BELONG HERE!"* screamed John. He had been quiet for quite awhile. They were definitely cutting the medication back. I got up and walked out of the room.

"Was that so hard? Now we get the hell out of here, or do you plan on making friends with all the rest of the nut cases in here? Are you going to stay long enough for little Miss Hot Pants to take a good run at the schizoid? This isn't the fucking Holiday Inn. Get a plan. Here is my plan: get out of here, get rid of Asshole and we have a life! Oh shit! Look at you! You're not going to be able to do it, are you?"

I went back in my room. I sat on my bed, my back against the wall, clutching my pillow and fighting the tears. Could I do it? Could I make it on my own? I tried to remember all the things Dr. Jurgens told me that would help me to live on my own. I had made a list once. Or had I? I meant to, one listing all my attributes. We had talked about my intelligence. How smart I was. I was pretty confident of that, most of the time. We talked about my ability to manage things. That was true, after all Christine had always taken care of the banking and the bills. We talked about my ability to make friends and socialize. Chris, Sally and Christine never lacked friends if they wanted them; that wasn't so important to Christine and never important to John. They talked about being able to support myself and get a job. That really worried me. I had blown two careers because of my behavior. Even that, Dr. Jurgens assured me, would work it out. It was so overwhelming to think about, so frightening. I felt so alone. Suddenly I wondered if living alone would feel any worse than this.

I wished that Rick could have really loved me. He hadn't even called since I had come to the hospital. When he had been unfaithful the first time and I had forgiven him, we had gotten on our knees and recommitted our lives to each other and to God. He had told me that I was the love of his life. I wanted to believe this so much but this didn't feel like being the love of anyone's life. I wondered what being the love of someone's life felt like. This was too hard to think about. I curled up and went to sleep.

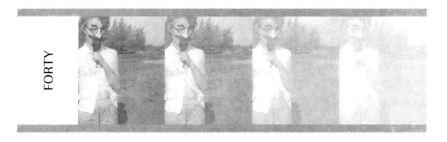

# FORTY

# We Have a Plan

Monday morning at the Villas was psychiatric consultation day. After breakfast I was summoned to what used to be the sunroom. It had glass on all four sides: two faced an outside courtyard where the nurses went to smoke; the other two faced inside toward the nurses' station and a hallway where patients, nurses or anyone else wandered all the time. It was kind of like being in a fishbowl and would be pretty uncomfortable if you craved privacy.

*How long have I been here?* I wondered as I walked into the room. I knew it had been at least five or six days—in actuality, it had been ten days. I forced a smile on my face. I really disliked this doctor. He liked to speak to my breasts reminding me of that old high school teacher I had found so mean and arrogant.

"Hello," he said, smiling directly at my breasts then quickly shifting his eyes to my face. "You're looking much better than the last time I saw you," he said, glancing quickly again at my breasts, then up again. "How you are feeling?"

"I am feeling better." I answered.

"How do you like the boobs, *PIG?*" John echoed in my head.

"Is the depression lifting? he asked.

"Yes, I think so." I answered.

"Let's get this over with, give the idiot what he wants!" John said.

"You have been seeing Dr. Jurgens?" he asked as he shuffled through the file.

"Yes, I have a couple of times," I answered.

"Enough already, get this clown out of here!" John snarled.

"That is helping?" another inane question from the shrink.

"For sure," I answered.

"'That is helping?' . . . What do you think she is going to say, idiot, freaking idiot!" John was unrelenting.

"You will continue to see him?" he asked.

"He needs to be slapped, get us out of here, DO IT NOW!"

"Yes, I will," I answered. "When do you think I can go home?"

"Have you been having any more thoughts of suicide?" he asked.

"Oh, here we go!" John continued. "This guy's a freaking idiot, laughable at best, even on his GOOD DAY! He has a bank account doubling by the minute. Give him what he wants so we can get the hell out of here!" John was livid.

It was time for Christine. I, Chris, could not deal with all this.

"Let me handle this," Christine popped in, "I will get us out of here."

*Please, no more! No more!* I thought. I was close to tears.

"You have to let me deal with this, or we will never get out of here. And no tears," Christine insisted.

"Then handle it!" John was very angry again.

Elizabeth soothed me, shushed John and let Christine take control. For all intents and purposes there had just been a very quick Board meeting! If the doctor had been paying attention he would have noticed the shiver and tilting of my head.

"No, there have been no more thoughts of suicide, I have been feeling very strong, I would like to go home," Christine replied.

"That might be a little soon. How things are for you at home, are you under a lot of stress there?" the doctor queried. He had my file so he should have known the answers to these questions.

"Yes, there are problems, but I have plans in place on how to deal with them," Christine answered calmly.

"What is your plan?" the doctor probed.

The Board had met. They had a plan. It was to take care of the immediate situation and handle this doctor and get out of the hospital. That meant Christine needed to be in charge.

"I have to leave my husband," Christine answered.

She heard John somewhere cheering and being told to be quiet by Elizabeth. It made her want to smile. No, no smiling not now, that would be counter-productive at this stage of the conversation in light of the fact that this "good doctor" didn't believe any of these other people existed.

Christine continued, "I cannot continue to live in my present circumstance." There, the words had been said out loud. Everyone had heard them. All the Directors had been there.

"Do you have a support system in place?" the doctor asked.

"I don't have the details worked out, but I have family and friends I can turn to," she answered. She was lying through her teeth. She didn't have any idea how she was going to go about any of this. She just wanted out of there. What she did know was how the hospital system worked: as soon as they thought you were no longer a threat to yourself or anyone else you were on your way home.

It was quite a performance by Christine—and it had worked. The doctor said, "Very well, I will prepare the paperwork and you will be free to go home by this evening."

By lunchtime the other patients knew I would be leaving. A few asked for my phone number, but you never give anyone your real number in these places, or reveal your last name, or tell them what town you are from. I handed my fake number out several times, wishing everyone the best, promising to call, promising to pray. It is all stuff you did and stuff you even meant on your first stay in one of these places, but you learned the ropes after a couple times around the psych ward. Did you really want any of these people showing up on your doorstep for Easter Sunday brunch?

All the other patients were still seated at the dining room table when Jake stood beside me, bent over and took my face gently in his big brown hand. Placing his cheek beside mine he said, for one last time, "Isn't this the whitest woman you ever saw?" He laughed that wonderful, deep, infectious laugh. When everyone had finally stopped laughing, he turned and started to walk away. Then he turned back toward me and said "White woman!" I realized in that second that he had never called me by my real name. "I'm still going to marry you someday!"

I smiled and nodded. Then he turned and continued down the hall. I watched him disappear into his room. I felt like crying. He hadn't asked for my number. Jake was wiser than that.

That evening I signed the discharge papers. It was all such a joke, such a farce. What had really been gained? I walked the long corridor out to the parking lot. Sitting in my car the words, "You would sooner be dead than alive with Rick" rang in my head. "But I am not strong enough to live alone," I said.

"Fuck—here we go! Yes you are! Let me handle this! Let Christine do this! Let Christine and me do this! Back out of it if you can't do it!" said John.

Christine said, "Yes! We can do it! We are smart enough! Social Services will help!"

"What about Cory? Where will we live?" I cried.

"We can stay! Kick him out! Make him leave! After all! It's your home, kick him out!" implored John.

"No I can't! What will I live on? I can't stay in Riverdale! I am too ashamed!" I was still crying.

"We can move! There's help. We can find help!" urged Christine.

"Can't! Just can't. I have to wait till Cory is out of school! It will be okay! It will be okay! It's not that bad! He's treating me okay!" I said.

"Right, where is hubby now? How has he been treating you okay? How much KY jelly are you going to have to use? How much humiliation, Chris, before the next suicide attempt?" asked Christine.

"Stop now! Stop! Stop! I can't hear this! I need to get home!" I said.

Before I knew it I was parked in front of the liquor store.

"No booze! Fuck the booze! Stop her!" said John.

"It's the only way she has of shutting you up. You're scaring her. Let me talk to her," said Christine.

John said, "This has to stop, we are never going to get out of there if she doesn't quit this! She has to leave him or she will kill us! He needs to die! Maybe that's the way out of this! She has to quit drinking! Why can't she see that? I will kill the useless bastard! Yes I will! I will KILL HIM!"

"She will kill us! He needs to die! She will kill us! He needs to die! She will kill us!" John was in a full rant. "If we don't kill him or get us out of there she will kill us!"

The words rebounded in my head like waves crashing against the rocks. I remembered a trip Rick and I had taken after Rose-anne had passed away. Mom and Dad had insisted we take their van and get away for awhile so we went to the Oregon coast. I had always loved the ocean. Why did I remember being there? It was February. The ocean was cold and rugged and powerful. The rocks had been so big. The ocean was so big, so strong. I had never seen anything that massive, that potent before. I could see myself, sitting on that huge grey rock, the waves pounding. I loved the way the mist stung my face. I didn't ever want to leave. I wanted to listen to the roar forever, feel the stinging on my skin forever. I wanted to be there now.

"She will kill us! He needs to die! She will kill us! He needs to die! She will kill us," John continued to rant.

"Where am I?"

"Liquor store."

"Get a bottle!"

"Get home!"

"Get Cory!"

"Psych ward! Jake!"

"Laughter!"

We Have a Plan                                    233

"Kill him! No! No!"

"Have a drink!"

"Stop the voices! Stop the voices! Get home! Get home! Get home! Get home!

"Stop the voices!"

"John is too mad this time!"

"Stop the voices! Stop the voices!"

"Have a drink!"

"Stop the voices!"

"Look after Cory!"

"Stop the voices!"

"Have a drink!"

The Directors were in a terrible state. No one knew what was going on. No one was in charge. It was a cacophony.

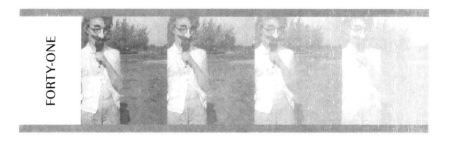

FORTY-ONE

# Long Days and Short Years

I had downed half a bottle of vodka on the drive home. It was one way to keep John quiet, at least it seemed to work on occasion. Somehow I made it home. My sisters had called the night before; I vaguely remembered talking to one or more of them. I passed out again and I woke up, luckily, in my own bed. My head pounded. I was clear enough to realize that I had a list of things to do. First, I needed to call Janet Schmidt to tell her that I was home and to thank her for looking after Cory. Next, I had to call the school and get a message to Cory to tell him to come home after school. Finally, I needed to get a hold of Rick's work and leave a message for him. I paused, wondering why I needed to bother with that.

The phone rang. It was Dr. Jurgens. "Hello Chris. I was just checking up on you. How are you doing now that you are home?"

"I am just fine," I said reassuringly. "I am so much better after my rest in the psych ward." The words seemed to bounce back at me like an echo.

"Excellent. Make sure to call if you need anything," he said.

I hung up and looked around my beautiful house. Now it seemed so cold, so unfeeling. I loved the color scheme, all the shades of blue, my favorite color. It had been the first time in my life that I had ever been involved in things like paint chips and recessed lighting. There had been dozens of decisions to make, from kitchen cupboard hardware, to the brand name and color of appliances. Everything was just the way I wanted it. We had done cool things like put a hidden sewing machine in the cupboards and a closeted laundry room on the main floor. There was a game room in the basement that Rick had finished himself. The carpeting had nice, thick padding and still looked brand new.

Decorating was the last thing on my mind now. I was tired; so much for the respite and realignment that the Villas was supposed to provide. I wasn't hysterical but I was sure not well.

No one was expecting me as they were not notified about my release. Rick was on the road. Craig, was away at college, and Cory was staying with our friends the Schmidt family, thank goodness. They had been an incredible blessing. I had gotten to know them through school and having their son in the children's program at my church. Their son was Cory's age, and he and Cory had always got along well. They were a farm family with horses, dogs, cats and hearts as big as all outdoors. Somehow they always understood when I was in trouble and Cory needed a place to be. I never had to explain, never had to worry, and always knew he would be looked after by them. Even more important was that they accepted him for who he was; something rare and wonderful in itself. They would take care of Cory. I knew that.

I sat down and wondered where the years had gone. The boys had grown so quickly. How much of that did I lose by being so sick? The marriage might have been awful but my boys were what really kept me going. They were so different from each other but such great kids in their own way.

Craig was such a determined young man. When he was in grade seven, for instance, he decided that there needed to be a Bible study for his age group. Taking matters into his own hands, he started one and he carried that on himself for two years. Sometimes he held it at the church; sometimes he arranged to have it at the school, regardless of what he had to encounter to get that done. Grade seven was also the year he came to me and told me he knew he would be going into the ministry—that would be his life's work. It would be. His path never changed.

Craig and I had a unique closeness for a mother and son. I had loved it when he had his friends over and they sat around the table and talked about all kinds of things that kids think about: from are there really aliens out there to what really did happen to the dinosaurs? I enjoyed being part of youth group functions, watching Craig in his element, watching him blossom and grow. It was great to spring him a day off from school and take him shopping to the Christian bookstore. I would get him the latest "in your face" T-shirt and more Christian rock music and posters. We would talk all the way home about how "really hard" it was to be a Christian. I would tell him how proud I was of him. I loved the times he would come and get me to listen to a special song he really liked, or the times something was bothering him and we would pray together.

He matured so quickly in every way, especially spiritually. He had started going away to Tumble River Bible Camp for a week in the summer as soon as he was old enough. When he was fourteen, they asked him to stay on as a counselor in training. He was actually too young for the program but if we gave our permission they would make an exception for him. He really wanted to do this so Rick and I agreed to let him stay for two more weeks. The two weeks turned into most of the summer and for all intents and purposes he never spent another summer at home.

Much different than Craig, Cory couldn't sit still. He loved being outside. He had a bubbly, outgoing, sometimes noisy personality and he got along with people of any age. He was also a boy's boy and treasured time spent with his dad, whether it was fishing or working alongside him. He was also fearless: one time, when he was only five or six years old, he walked right into the middle of a herd of cattle. Rick found him in the corral with a dozen cows around him looking at him like he was a little alien. He had some grass in his hand and was feeding them; he was so small any one of them could have stepped on him without noticing.

The years we lived on the farm he spent many hours riding on tractors with the neighbors around our home. Cory's hyperactivity and lack of understanding of consequences led him on many adventures though it was something he eventually outgrew. He had been a handful but could melt my heart with a smile, like the day I looked out the window at my garden and the row of fourteen-foot tall sunflower plants were chopped down each at exactly the same height. I saw Cory walking away with a small camping axe. When I went out and asked him what was up, he gave me that smile and told me he was playing lumberjack. I could hardly get angry at him—but from then on, I stored the axe in a spot that was just a little too high for him to reach. One thing I knew for sure: life with Cory never boring.

I often wondered if Craig or Cory knew, if they had picked up on anything—my illness, the marital troubles. We were the faithful Sunday churchgoers and the Wednesday night Bible students but then things started slipping so badly even though I fought so hard. When the memories started coming back and I started to come to grips with the "voices" was also the time Rick fell off the wagon and refused to go back to AA. I had and still was searching desperately within Christian circles for help. There was no peace, none, no amount of prayer would bring it back. It was like there had been this incredible shift in the universe and everything was off balance and I was in this horrible fight to get this lined up again. The marital problems alone would have been enough to send most families over the edge, let alone what I was dealing with. There had been no peace in my head for years—how had that affected my kids?

I thought about Craig and Cory felt incredible guilt. I felt like I had abandoned ship, I didn't have the time, didn't have the energy, not like I had in the beginning. Craig was so strong, had such incredible faith, it had been easy to let him look after himself. He was out of the house now and, after all was said and done, he was all right. When I let him counsel at Tumble River Camp that first summer I knew that part of my decision was so that he couldn't see what really was happening at home. The goal was:

Keep Rick away in the truck as much as possible; keep Craig in as many Christian activities as he wanted so he didn't notice; keep Cory on Ritalin. Maybe, just maybe, I could keep the show on the road, at least until the boys were on their own.

Craig was in college now and loved it, he also arranged to work summers at a remote Bible camp. I was so proud of him. *Perhaps I can stick this out till he graduates.*

A voice jolted me out of my reverie. "What? Has to be now!" It was John. "Has to be now, you can't live with that useless piece of skin anymore!"

He was always calling Rick a useless piece of skin. It was one of John's favorite expressions. He was so crude. I wished he would just be quiet and leave me alone.

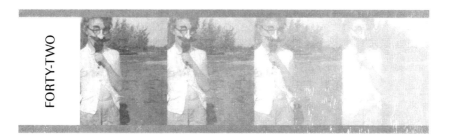

FORTY-TWO

## *Searching for Wildflowers*

The Board quieted down after I had arrived home from the Villas, sobered up, and eventually settled in again. I got a lot of sleep. I would wake with Cory get him breakfast send him off to school, go back to bed till noon, make him lunch, sleep a couple more hours till he got home again and then go to bed when he did at night. Rick was away working as usual. When he got home that weekend he took Cory on a father/son fishing trip through the church. Even though I was ostracized, several of the men remained in contact with Rick, most of whom had been friends of his since childhood. They always included him on their outings, especially the father/son activities. I slept another day and woke up Saturday morning feeling fantastic and full of energy.

The next day was yard work day. The perennial flower garden needed weeding and by lunchtime that was done. I decided it needed more wildflowers so after lunch I set out for a drive to see what I could find. It was early June and the lady slippers were in bloom and with any luck the tiger lilies may have started. I would be back before Cory got out of school.

Lady slippers are my favorite flower. They are so perfectly formed they their name is so appropriate. Two different kinds grow here locally: the big fat ones and the smaller more delicate ones, each shaped in the image of a slipper. I hoped I was not too late for the blooming season. I drove past the farming area I had been raised in. It didn't even phase me that I had to go right past the old school where Mom had taken me and my sisters to dances, past the farm of the people who had told me about my dad, and the incident where one of the twin boys was killed. There were no flashbacks, just a relaxing wonderful drive in the country searching for beautiful wildflowers.

When I was younger this was my backyard. As a girl I went hunting and snowmobiling in this area with my dad and then continued the tradition later on with my husband. None of that mattered now. Today I was looking for lady slippers. This was beautiful countryside with mixed forest: tamarack, spruce, poplar, and birch trees, and cranberry bushes. There were a multitude of wildflowers: bluebells, Indian paintbrush, fireweed and wild daisies. I drove and inhaled the beauty while I watched for lady slippers, waiting to see their little yellow heads in among the lush green undergrowth.

It was a quiet, beautiful day. Unlike the madness of the few days before, there was real peace in my head today. *Why can't every day be like this?* I asked myself, but quickly moved past that thought to simply enjoy the beauty surrounding me.

There was the first one. My heart began to thump. I slowed the car down and turned off the main road onto the next side road, driving very slowly. I knew what to watch for, where they grew. Sure enough, their little yellow heads started to appear more often. I smiled, yellow was a happy color. I drove until I felt I had found just the right spot. I stopped the car and walked into the forest. I was not disappointed. It was a good year. I found a nice grouping of eight and I dug them out with a spade, being careful to take enough of the surrounding environment so that I did not disturb the root system. It was actually illegal to remove them from their natural state, but I never felt guilty because I treated them with such reverence. I had already successfully transplanted some before so knew the procedure.

Back at home the small backyard was beginning to take shape. The construction of the house and the two-car garage had left very little room in the back for much other than a flower garden. It had been fun. I had loved picking the kinds of flowers, selecting perennials and herbs, Tiny Tim tomatoes, and other plants for eating. I even added some cool stepping stones I had hand-painted myself. I had taken great pride in this plot of land. The dark rich soil smelled good as I finished pushing it in around the lady slippers. I thought, *I hope they like it here.*

With the garden tools put away in the garage I walked toward the back of the property. A warm breeze blew the smell of burnt wood up into my nostrils. There was still a pile of salvaged articles from the house fire that had happened only the previous year piled in the back; things we could use but never got the smoke smell out of.

It had been a wonderful couple of days; quiet, peaceful, even productive days. I so wished I would have more like them: tranquil days where I had a purpose. I felt normal. Days like these gave me something I had not had in a long time—maybe ever. Days like these gave me hope.

# FORTY-THREE

# The Final Discussion

"You would sooner be dead than live with him." I kept hearing the words. What would it be like? I didn't love him. I never had, not really. I had been in love with the *idea* of having a mate who would love and take care of me. That had never happened; in fact it was exactly the opposite. I always had to look after him. Now Rick was on a mission to convince me that his infidelity was mostly, if not all, my fault. He seemed incapable of acknowledging any of my pain. The Directors were about to have their final discussion on the matter.

Rick and I were in the sunroom one evening, the pretty little sunroom, designed for days of relaxed reading and nights of serenity and stargazing. We were having another one of our discussions on why I couldn't just put this last infidelity behind me and move on.

"You just don't get it, you don't get how badly this hurts!" I was close to tears out of complete frustration. I continued, "Why can't you even *try* to understand how I feel?"

Looking at me, he matter-of-factly said, "I don't know why you're so upset, they were just prostitutes."

Something snapped in my head. I found myself screaming, loud enough for neighbors several blocks away to have heard. I suddenly felt like I was defending all women. It was so strange. I looked at him like I had never seen him before, like I had no idea who he was.

"They were *women!*" I yelled, "Someone's daughter, mother, sister, friend; what do you mean they were *just* prostitutes?" I walked back into the main house, not giving him a chance to answer. The subject was over. He had said it all.

John jumped on that opportunity, "He will never change. This is not going to get better. Do you really think he is going to treat you any better? Kick his ass out, or let's get out now. He's too fucking stupid to change. Cripes! Thinking that shit is one thing, but saying it out loud? That's a stupid man; we deserve better!"

"You have to go with this, we can do this, we are good at reflexology, we can do that anywhere," said Christine. "We can move to Merrimore and you could take your clients from here with you."

A soft voice seldom heard from but always there said, "We can do this together." It was Elizabeth. "We are getting stronger all the time. We need to work together and not be so afraid."

"We could?" I asked, and it dawned on me that there was, indeed, some hope. "What about Sally?" I asked.

"What about me? It would be so awesome on our own! I wouldn't be trouble, honest." giggled Sally.

"We *have* to take Cory with us. Cory *needs* to come with us," I said.

And so the dialogue to finally move away from Rick had started in earnest. I was so excited. I couldn't wait to call Dr. Jurgens. There was peace in my head, like the Directors had come to an agreement. I was looking forward to my next appointment with him so everyone could be there.

Then the phone rang and once again everything had to change. It was Craig. He was away at Bible camp, having finished another year at Bible college, through which he was halfway to getting his degree. "Mom, I've got some great news," he said. "I met a young lady at camp, Lilly, a counselor. We got to be really serious this summer. More than serious, really, we are deeply in love. I've asked her to marry me, Mom, and she said *yes!*"

"Oh, Craig, that is fantastic news!" I said. Craig went on to tell me that she was from a city close to the Bible school. They had it all figured out. She had just graduated from grade twelve, so she planned to work for the next year. He was working part-time and going to school. They would get married the following spring. She would continue to work while he finished his fourth year of Bible college. Needless to say, I was in shock, but they seemed very set in what they wanted. They had already met with her parents and Craig had gone so far as to ask her father for her hand in marriage. While I was concerned that they were so young, as Rick and I had been, I also knew my son. Craig had always been the epitome of level-headedness and she was the perfect, pretty Christian girl. So in ten months Craig and Lilly were going to be married and that was that.

Now this made little to no difference to John, but it made all the difference in the world to me, Chris. I had maintained this wonderful show for this long. I was going to keep on the good face until after the wedding. I couldn't bear the thought of embarrassing Craig and for that matter Cory who had a couple more years left in high school. Deep down, I really wanted him to have that behind him before I dismantled what was left of the marriage. John wasn't buying it. He accused me of looking for an excuse, of being a coward. The battle in the boardroom was back on. It would get even crazier in the months to come, as booze became a bigger player on the scene.

Sessions with Dr. Jurgens were becoming very animated. In the past it had taken much coaxing to get different alters to appear, now there was often a competition to see who would get to speak.

Christine would often appear first, saying that the trip to see Dr. Jurgens was one long debate among the Board to see who would be the one to be present. The debate was futile anyway as it seemed to make little or no difference once she was there. The switching between personalities was rapid fire, like when you change your mind about something.

As different as the alters were, they did all have one thing in common: they all trusted Doug implicitly—even John. At this point I had been in therapy a couple of years and had made a lot of progress, though to someone from the outside looking in, it might not have appeared so. Dr. Jurgens had been very positive as he worked to gain the confidence of each of the alters. That, of course, took a lot of time, and understandably so. My psyche had created them in part because there was no one I could go to for help—no one I felt I could rely upon. Because of these trust issues, ingrained also in the Board, the healing process was long and arduous.

Dr. Jurgens avoided the use of the word "integration" because it was too intimidating for us. Instead he focused on respect for each alter and recognition and full acceptance of how each had played a part in my overall survival. He encouraged a healthy dialogue between us and would point out when one alter was doing something to upset another. For instance, when John was stealing he would tell him how much it upset Chris. Eventually, each individual alter came to accept and respect the others and without ever using the label of "integration."

At one point John had been sure the mission was to destroy him but now, even for John, this was a place to be heard. The other alters wouldn't listen to him but here in this room, with this doctor, he had found someone who would acknowledge him and pay attention to what he had to say. To John, if ever there was a time to get his message through it was now, especially with Sally being able to have so much time cavorting with Rick.

One day John was in the room at therapy and he was upset. He sat straight up with his back pushed hard against the chair, feet flat on the floor, legs spread with his arms crossed in front of his chest.

"Good to see you John," Doug greeted him.

"Thanks," said John.

"It looks like you might have something on your mind," Dr. Jurgens said.

"Do you know what's going on? Have you any idea? This is going to put us back in the looney bin, this *will* take us down," John accused.

"You're going to have to be more specific, I think I know what you're talking about—I got a letter from Elizabeth—but you tell me. What's happening?" Dr. Jurgens asked.

"Miss Hot Pants has been out and is doing Hubby. Can you wrap your brain around that shit? Oh, yeah! Doing him all right! Think I am going to keep letting that happen, and the thing is Chris doesn't know! Think she will be able to handle that now? No way! There is *no* fucking way! We had a plan! We were leaving him. Chris will kill us if we don't stop her!

"What do you mean, about Miss Hot Pants?" the doctor asked.

"Sally, who do you think?" John was getting impatient.

"Why doesn't Chris know?" Dr. Jurgens asked.

"What? I don't know, but she doesn't. It's the booze maybe, or the pills, maybe Elizabeth is looking after her, but it's only a matter of time and when she finds out you know she won't be able to handle it. She will kill us! It will be suicide time again. You have to do something," John said. "Chris will become suicidal and kill us all." John warned.

"Is Chris here? Can I talk to her?" Dr. Jurgens asked.

Shiver and tilt; another Director was arriving. She remained sitting straight in the chair, but crossed her legs at the ankles and placed her hands one on top of the other in her lap. She leaned a little forward and looked directly into Dr. Jurgens' face, smiling.

Dr. Jurgens did a quick recovery, for this was a very rare event. It was not Chris who had come but Elizabeth.

"Hello," he said, "I know you have been helping."

"Thanks," she said, "You know they don't mean to lie or hide things, it's just the way they are. They are so afraid, especially Chris—and even Christine and John. Oh, he pretends to be big and brave, but sometimes they are just afraid, you must forgive them."

"You have been around a long time, Elizabeth; you have seen a lot," Dr. Jurgens said, "What has that been like for you?"

"I haven't minded," Elizabeth said. She leaned back against the chair, crossing and uncrossing her hands in her lap. She smiled, then leaned forward again and said in a soft voice, "You mustn't give up on them; we mustn't *ever* give up."

"Is Chris in trouble right now Elizabeth? How serious is this?" he asked.

"I think she will be okay; it is so important to her that everything stays perfect for Craig's wedding, but she is drinking way too much and I am very concerned about that," Elizabeth replied.

"What is happening with John and his criminal behavior?" he asked.

Dr. Jurgens was going to make use of this opportunity while he had it. Elizabeth was the "truth center" of the system. She knew what was happening and she held the memories, but unlike the others she wasn't always in control. Unlike the others she had nothing to hide nor fear, her role nevertheless was to protect.

She sat quietly pondering the question. Elizabeth would not be rushed. She was more than comfortable in her own skin. She was levelheaded and weighed her answers and the consequences of them carefully.

"You might consider asking him about some other things he has been up to," Elizabeth replied.

"Thank you, I will. What about Sally? John tells me Sally has been around a lot lately." Dr. Jurgens had decided to follow another path.

"Yes, you know that from my letters. It's very upsetting, she means no harm, sweet girl, but you know how Chris gets about all that," Elizabeth responded, "and that makes John very angry."

"I really think it would be a good thing if I could talk to Chris before you leave today, Elizabeth. Is there any way you can help with that, or can you talk to her for me?" Dr. Jurgens pressed.

Shiver and tilt. This time she crossed her legs and rested her arms on the arms of the chair. She remained sitting straight in the chair but with less formality though obviously very much in control.

"Hi," she said in a strong, clear voice. Christine had arrived.

"Hi," Dr. Jurgens responded. "This is great, good to have you here Christine."

"She can't deal with any of this now. Why are you insisting on talking to her? What are you hoping to accomplish?" Christine asked with a good measure of animosity in her voice.

"Is that why you are here Christine? So I can talk to her through you, like we have in the past? Because that would be great, and you're right she can't deal with this right now without your help. I am very concerned about that, but you know she is going to find out what has been going on. That is going to happen, one way or another. You can't stop that. Christine, it is happening to her, too. She could suddenly be there in the middle of sex with Rick, then what happens to her? Elizabeth tells me John has been engaged in some more criminal behavior. We have to warn her about that, too. She is going to find out about this, in fact I suspect she already has some idea about this stuff already. You all have to be working together," Dr. Jurgens pushed Christine.

"That's not what Elizabeth said!" Christine shot back.

"No you're right. She said I should ask him what he's been up to. Are you going to tell me that means he hasn't been up to something? Chris has to know what has been happening and has to get help for the drinking, because if she doesn't and if she is allowed to hide, this will cave in on her and then something *terrible* could happen here. Is she there now, Christine?" Dr. Jurgens continued to push.

Christine squirmed uncomfortably in her chair for a second but quickly regained her composure.

"She is here, isn't she? Can she hear us?" Dr. Jurgens probed Christine.

"She's here, she's very afraid," Christine responded. "She can hear us."

"Chris, I am glad you're here. You're safe here. We can talk through Christine. That's not a problem. I am worried about you. We need to look after you, and we need to talk about some things that have been happening at home. Can you talk to me?" Doug asked.

Shiver and tilt. I crossed my legs up under my body, hung my head down onto my chest and started to cry. Doug placed a hand on one of my shaking shoulders and handed me a tissue. I sat that way for a few minutes, letting the tears fall on my lap, not even trying to wipe them away with the tissue. There were no words. It was quiet except for my crying.

Finally the tears stopped and I looked up. "I am so tired. I need this to stop. I can't talk about leaving right now, there's the wedding . . . after the wedding . . . I can't talk about leaving now, please!" I said, crying again.

"We don't need to talk about that, no problem. I want to talk about the drinking. I received a letter about it and have been talking to Elizabeth and she's worried about the drinking," he said.

"It's not that bad, she worries too much. I like to drink to get to sleep. I don't even do that much anymore. It's not always me you know, sometimes it's Sally. She takes us to parties. It's no big deal, I'm fine, Sally hasn't even been that bad lately. It's no big deal. I just do it sometimes to get some sleep, really." I protested.

"Let's talk about Sally then. You say she hasn't been doing the party thing, what do you mean?" he asked.

"I mean I haven't ended up in a hotel room out of town anywhere, that's what," I replied.

"Do you think she may be doing other things?" Dr. Jurgens asked.

I got a very strange look on my face. "Good grief, what's that supposed to mean?" I asked.

A sick feeling started to come over me as the realization of what he might be talking about settled in. Not that this was a new situation. It certainly wouldn't be the first time Sally had surfaced for a while and been Rick's lover. In fact at times in the past that had been an unsaid but just the same very mutually agreed on arrangement between the members of the Board. Why wouldn't Sally handle that part of the marriage considering who she was and what she did? But times had changed. There had been a whole new consensus; the Board couldn't accept the disrespect dealt out in the marriage. It had become unacceptable at any level for them to stay involved with him, so for Sally to step in at this point and be involved with him sexually wasn't going to go unnoticed, regardless of the fact that Sally was just being Sally and had no malicious intent. This would serve to bring the rest of the alters together in a different way. A way that was stronger and more focused albeit, very inexperienced.

"Oh, that makes sense," I said slumping further in my chair. "She does things I won't do; no wonder things have been better the last few weekends. Sally is *doing* him!" I started to cry again. "I hate him, I really do hate him, but I have a son getting married. I have made it this far; I will make it until after that, I have to!" I said.

My eyes were red and I felt tired and beaten. I took a tissue and wiped my eyes, untangled my legs and made a half-hearted effort at composure.

"Doug, my life is out of control," I said. "It's all about sex! It's always been about *sex!* My entire life has revolved around it! It started with my dad before I could even spell it and it has controlled my life ever since. That's a lot of control. It should be mine. I want that control. It needs to be mine." The tears pooled in my eyes again.

"Help me, I can't give up. Someday, the control has to be mine, Doug, I have to keep going until after Craig's wedding," I cried.

The session time was nearly over and Dr. Jurgens needed to make sure we were all going to be strong enough to go home.

"How are you going to deal with Sally?" he asked.

Shiver and tilt. "I think we are fine, it wasn't as big a deal as she made it out. You know how she likes to be the drama queen." Christine responded.

"Are you going to be able to get everyone home?" he asked.

"I think so, seems pretty quiet. The trick will be to get them past the liquor store. If I can do that, half the battle is won. I will do my best," she answered.

"We have an appointment next week and open phone calls anytime. I am trusting you to take everyone home safely. Is there anyone you think I should or need to talk to before you leave?" he asked.

Christine shook her head no.

"Then before you go," he said, "I want to thank everyone, it was great to talk to you all, let's all talk again soon and, Elizabeth, thanks for the letters." He gave her a hug before he walked her out.

And so the sessions went, hour after hour, week after week as the Directors sought to work together, sought to reach new understandings of who they had been, who they were and who they were to become. They all had come to an unspoken agreement about Craig's wedding. John had even seemed to be on board and had been leaving Chris alone in so far as he hadn't been harassing her about leaving. In fact, he had been very quiet of late. Dr. Jurgens had tried to find out about any further criminal activity and hadn't been able to turn up anything new, and I was comfortable with that. I had searched the house looking for stolen credit cards, extra cash, or anything else suspicious and hadn't found anything, so I assumed there hadn't been anything new in the works. Sally was still arriving the odd weekend and spending it with Rick, but I had even come to terms with that for the time being. I saw it as a blessing, as warped as that might seem. I was still drinking and I knew it was too much, especially with the amount of pills I was taking, but I loved the escape it gave me.

Occasionally it still overwhelmed me and I did make use of the provision to check into the local hospital for a couple of days—a couple of days of total escape to get some rest and tackle life again.

Craig had a beautiful May wedding. He was so handsome and Lily made a lovely bride. They looked truly happy. I had made sure to take my little white pills that morning. I would do nothing to spoil his wedding day, and yet all I could think was it had already been spoiled. The Christian family he had grown up with and believed in never really existed.

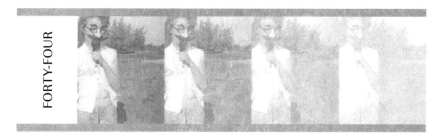

# FORTY-FOUR

# The End, for Real

It was exactly a month after Craig's wedding when Rick, Cory and I went with Rick's sister and her husband to a car show one Friday evening in a neighboring town. We came back to our house and played a couple of card games. I liked these members of Rick's family and it was actually a very pleasant time; nothing dramatic had happened.

At about 11:00 PM, after our company left, I went into my typical pre-bedtime routine: tranquillizers and vodka. Three hours later I packed a suitcase and wrote Rick this note:

> Rick:
>
> I am leaving. I can't do this anymore. I will let you know where I am in a couple days so Cory won't worry. I want him with me. Don't even try to get me back. IT IS OVER.
>
> Christine

I got in my car, withdrew a thousand dollars from the bank, and drove to Regency, a city three hours away.

Just like that it was over—after all the fights, the negotiations, the failed reconciliations. My marriage of twenty-nine years ended on an ordinary evening. Though its demise had been coming for years the final gasp happened spontaneously. I had no plans and I had no clue where I was going to go next. All I knew for sure was that I would *not* be going back to Riverdale.

I stayed in Regency until Monday morning. I decided that I would live in Merrimore, the town I was in when I found out my house had burned down. When I got there, I went to Social Services and asked for help. I told them I didn't have a job and couldn't work. I also told them I couldn't live with my husband any longer. I called Dr. Jurgens from their office and he confirmed what I had told them. By that afternoon I'd been placed in a light-housekeeping suite in a local motel where I could stay until I found a place to rent.

With this much of my life in order I called Rick. "Where are you? I have been worried sick. When are you coming home?" he asked.

"Didn't you get my note?" I asked.

There was silence on the other end of the phone. "Yeah, but I thought once you sobered up you would come back," was his reply.

"I am sober, Rick," I said, shaking my head. "I am not coming back, not ever!" I said defiantly. I heard the words. *They* heard the words: John, Christine, Sally and Elizabeth all heard *the words*. This time they *knew* it was true. It was finally over.

"I am in Merrimore and I am looking for a place to rent," I said. "We need to talk about Cory."

"What do you think you're doing to this family *now?*" Rick asked. "Isn't this about enough? Come home when you sober up," he said as he hung up.

Part of what he said was true; though I was sober now I had spent most of the weekend drunk in Regency. I had a hell of a headache to prove it. I couldn't really blame Rick for not taking me seriously. This was going to take some time to sink in even for me. I couldn't help but think of how many times he had told me I could never make it on my own—I'd actually lost count. And hell,

*I* didn't know how I was going to make it on my own—but damn it anyway, I knew I was.

I was forty-eight years old, had a suitcase full of clothes, about $800 cash, my '88 Oldsmobile and felt optimistic for the first time in years.

I was a woman on a mission. Within two days I had found an apartment and signed a lease. It was a tiny two-bedroom apartment, but cute and clean, with a funky balcony that overlooked a park. I loved it. I could move into it in two weeks and two of my sisters from Alberta were going to come and help me.

I took very little of the new furniture that we had bought for our house after the fire. It was too big and wouldn't fit, plus I didn't want to upset Cory any more than necessary. My son had decided he was going to stay with his dad for the time being. It was the best for Cory until I could get settled in and adjusted. It was June so, since school was out, Rick often took him trucking with him. Rick promised—and he did uphold it—that he would work harder at being home when school was back in session. Cory would eventually come to live with me and finish grade twelve.

So instead of all the beautiful furniture I left behind, I furnished the apartment with the rumpus-room furnishings from our basement; things I had purchased at yard sales and auctions. Those material things didn't matter. What was important was being free and making sure I had room for Cory when he came to stay with me.

When I called Craig and told him about my move he was very upset. He kept asking if there wasn't any way I would reconsider and look at this as just a separation time, a time to heal and move forward. I said kindly but firmly, "No Craig, I can't." It was a difficult thing because I knew Rick was telling the boys that he very much wanted me back and was hoping and praying that given some time I would come back to my senses and to him. He had convinced them that we could be the happy family again. It really made me look like a mentally deranged home-wrecker and he the hero trying the salvage the sinking ship. But I was resolute and I know that deep down the boys understood even if they didn't want to.

A couple of weeks after I had been in the apartment Rick called and asked if he could stop in. He had some of my things he wanted to drop off and wanted to talk to me. It sounded fishy but I agreed.

"The apartment looks nice," he said, trying to make small talk. His clothes were all rumpled and he looked like he hadn't been sleeping well.

"Thanks," I replied, hoping he would leave soon.

"I want to try and win you back," he said, "I want us to date."

I wasn't sure I heard him, but John had. There was a terrible fuss in my head. He might as well have pointed a gun at me. I suddenly felt so threatened. "If you can't handle this, I can!" John shouted.

"It's okay, were all here. It's okay." They were all there, the entire Board of Directors. No one person was in charge. They were all in charge as a group, a united front. Everyone agreed on this decision. It was a rare and wonderful moment in time.

"I want a chance to win you back, I want us to date again, you are the love of my life," Rick continued.

I looked at him, looking so pathetic, with his empty words. *Empty words from an empty man,* I thought. I got up from the kitchen chair and walked to the door. I opened it as I calmly said, "I am never coming back. Nothing you can say or do is going to change that. Stop trying and stop giving the boys false hope; it's not fair to them. The sooner we get on with our lives the better. There's too much pain here to go back, so what we need to is start again and move on."

Rick remained in his chair staring at me. "You're really going to do this, you're really going to fuck our family," he said, anger now fairly seeping from him. "You are one cold-hearted bitch!"

I held the door open wider saying, "Funny, only a minute ago I was the love of your life . . . You need to leave now." I held the door open for him; he wasn't moving. I said, "Now!" and I opened the door all the way and it hit the wall. This time he complied, with his proverbial tail tucked between his legs. I added, "If you need to talk to me about the boys I am here anytime, but otherwise we have nothing to talk about, Rick. Start over!"

He was gone. I closed the door.

After Rick left I sat on the balcony in the hot July sun. It felt so good on my face. Wow, I had been strong. It had felt good. It had felt good not to have everyone yelling inside my head.

We had been married for nearly three decades, most of my adult life. What now? Not going back, I knew that. So for now I would just sit in the sun on my balcony overlooking the park.

My mind wandered, eyes closed. I thought about the sun in Florida when we had been there on our anniversary trip—the vacation paid for by John and one of his crime sprees. The sun felt different there: hotter and more intense. The Florida Keys fascinated me. The car trip on the Overseas Highway made me feel like I was driving across the ocean. We had taken a fishing trip off of Key West into the Gulf of Mexico and around into the Atlantic. The color of the ocean was so blue. I leaned back in my chair and could feel the breeze coming off the Atlantic; it had been a wonderful experience. I hoped I could go back someday. That had been a happy time, hadn't it? It had been quiet in my head then. All the other trips during my marriage flashed in my head—the trips to California, driving down the Pacific Coast from Vancouver all the way to Mexico; through the redwood forests and the rugged rocky coastline.

It was all so confusing, like watching someone else who had lived a dozen different lives already. It was getting too hot in the sun so I went back inside. My head ached. Was that from the sun? Perhaps I hadn't eaten yet. I tried to remember. *Who is this person? You're pathetic,* I thought to myself; *you can't even remember if you have eaten.*

I checked the calendar and the clock and my list beside it. Was it today Rick had been to visit? That seemed a long time ago already. There was nothing on the list to take care of. Everything's good until Thursday. I had another appointment with Dr. Jurgens on Thursday.

Unbelievable, I thought. Where was the super woman who juggled a dozen things at a time? Suddenly I felt like I was in a foreign land without a road map. I felt lost and confused, nothing was familiar. Everything became overwhelming, even the idea of preparing a real meal was too daunting a task now. That brought with it a host of memories of many, many huge meals I had put together, some with very little notice. It had not been unusual in the least to have over a dozen people for Sunday dinner and have everything on the table homemade from the soup to the buns to the apple pie for dessert. Rick had a huge family: seven sisters and three brothers with dozens of nieces, nephew and cousins. They didn't all live in our hometown but it seemed like there was always someone visiting. We also liked to entertain and often invited folks over after church. That sort of thing was encouraged among the congregation. I spent a lot of time maintaining a clean, pleasant home and a deep freeze ready for any occasion. I, Chris, enjoyed cooking and baking and did a lot of it. Now I wondered could I make myself some homemade vegetable soup? Maybe if I made a list, right, a list.

I became aware of my head aching again. *Wheel of Fortune* was coming on the television. That meant it was 5:00 PM. It was definitely time to have something to eat. I opened the cupboard door. Thank God for canned soup. What kind would I have tonight? Then I opened the fridge door for something to drink. *Coors! Coors Light! Right on, Sally's favorite brand of beer. Forget the soup!*

Sally cracked a beer and I opened a can of soup. Now there was awareness among the alters of the others coming and going and without being in a confining home relationship. They just came and went and came and went in a fluid motion. The beer was down the hatch and another one open before the soup was even warm. Sally started a bath. She then went to the closet to decide what to wear for her night out. I tossed some fragrant lavender oil in the tub and lit a couple vanilla scented candles. I turned the soup off and Sally opened another beer. The headache was gone, replaced with a wonderful sense of warmth and well-being. I slipped into the tub of hot bath water. It felt great on my skin; I loved how my skin felt, soft and alive. It was such a strange thing, to lie in a hot tub of water and smell the different smells around me. The scented candles and the lavender mixed to create a wonderful relaxing aroma. I felt safe and sexy. Safe and sexy, that was a very strange combination, for me at least, couldn't be, could it? This was a far cry from holding my face in a bath towel, like another lifetime away. It must be the beer. *Yes, that had to be it,* I thought.

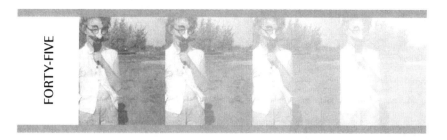

# FORTY-FIVE

# But We Look Good

So much confusion, I tried to shake it away. Sally had been in bars all over the province, but never in this town, only half an hour from where we had lived the past twenty-five years. The other alters had kept that kind of activity away from here: first, to protect Craig and Cory and second, because I had been raised in a family where outside appearances were paramount. As long as we *looked* good to the outside world, we *were* good. After all, I had the wonderful perfect Christian family to portray. It didn't seem necessary to do that anymore.

Sally walked right into that bar like she owned it and pissed off every woman in it immediately. It didn't take long before the first drink was sent over to her and the first man was hitting on her. Of course it wouldn't be only one drink and one man.

The party scene embraced Sally with open arms and she rushed in headfirst. Within a few short weeks she was completely out of control. Nothing had prepared us for what was out here. My new body image and not having any restraints was a ticking time bomb. The men loved me, and Sally's views on sex meant lots of sleeping around.

Even though my attitude had changed a lot I still wasn't ready to accept this and so there was constant turmoil going on between me—Chris—and Sally. That being said, the booze and Sally left me with very little to say. Sally would get dressed to go out, I would change her clothes. I would decide *no drinking tonight*, Sally would order one. Sally would invite a man over, I would ask him to leave.

Three months after leaving my husband, Dr. Jurgens and the Directors had agreed a rest was needed. This living alone had hit like a tidal wave. Never before did they have such complete freedom and as much as some were enjoying it, especially Sally, it was very scary to Chris. So back to the psych ward I went.

This time the admitting psychiatrist believed in the DID diagnosis so I didn't have to fudge that information. I still had to go through the standard drill. Was I having suicidal thoughts? When had they started? Had I attempted suicide recently, and did I have a plan? I gave the appropriate answers to get the admission I needed and once again found myself in a little room looking up at the wooden ceiling.

When *had* the suicidal thoughts started? I thought about that while I was staring at that ceiling. Maybe the week before when I was waiting for the results from the sexually transmitted disease tests I had taken. It made me sick to think about the number of men I had been with. Sally never worried about protected sex. Sally never worried about anything. Where was John these days or Elizabeth? Was this supposed to be the integrated life? *I can't work, my son's not even living with me anymore, but I can party. Oh yeah, this is a good thing. Oh, but we look good. That's always important; keep your make-up on and your hair done. This is insanity, just a different variety.* I hugged my pillow and waited for the drug-induced sleep to take over.

Dr. Jurgens had told me so many times to look at this as a healing time. Man that irked me. I couldn't remember anyone in my family ever being on social assistance. Since I could not stay employed because of my mental condition I was entitled to Canada Permanent Disability Pension, and received a rate based on Rick's and my combined salary when we had been together. It was really barely enough to live on so family and friends helped out. Still, that just wasn't supposed to happen. You worked and supported yourself.

Dr. Jurgens reminded me again and again not to feel ashamed or guilty about this. I was the victim here, right from when I was a little girl; that the things I was experiencing had been set in motion way back then. This was not my fault. I would replay those words again and again, but sometimes it just didn't make any sense. The whole thing just didn't make any sense. Why couldn't I make it work? He kept reassuring me that I would heal and I would become a working participating member of society again. He told me I had everything I needed to do that. He told me that there was no shame in letting people help. I wanted to believe that and sometimes I did. He told me over and over again about my intelligence, my creativity, and my charismatic and flamboyant personality. He told me that he could see a day when I would put my mind to something and there would be no stopping me. Then he would add, "But you have to get a hold of the drinking. I am afraid of your drinking. What a shame for you to get this far and then have something like alcohol take you out. You have to watch the booze!"

It was becoming quieter in my head. There was a lot less noise. John wasn't involved in criminal activity and that was a huge relief. John had mounted his wave of criminal activity in the first place because he wanted to bring attention to the fact that Chris was being taken advantage of. He rectified the situation by getting revenge, in this case through theft. Once he felt I didn't need that kind of protection anymore, then he didn't need to seek the attention that way and the activity stopped. "Does that mean I am becoming integrated?" I had asked Dr. Jurgens when he had come to see me on the ward.

"I am not sure about that," he had said. "Tell me about you and Sally."

"She has to settle down, that's crazy, she's out of control," I replied.

There was the familiar shiver and tilt. "Oh please, Chris is having a blast," Sally said with a giggle. "She just won't admit it, especially with the new boyfriend. She's never had such a good time, shaking that sweet booty all over the place." She giggled again and said, "Wow—hey—how you been? She doesn't let me talk to you much—you know why? Damn hospital. Hey, how long do you suppose we are going to be here this time? Do you suppose that good-looking guy Gary is here?"

"Good to see you, Sally. Chris is pretty worried about the partying and the unprotected sex," said Dr. Jurgens.

Sally giggled again, "She worries too much. She is having fun. She hasn't danced this much in years. She loves to dance and I told you to ask her about the boyfriend," she said giggling some more.

Shiver and tilt. "Was Sally here, what did she say?" I, Chris, joined them.

"Yes, she was," Dr. Jurgens replied. "She says you are having a better time than you are letting on and I should ask you about a new boyfriend."

Shaken and embarrassed I searched for words. I had been blindsided by Sally, that's for sure. Time and time again this was how the Board worked, leaking information about each other to the doctor, which he would bring back to them and they would then process together. This was often Elizabeth's and John's area, seldom Sally's, however this seemed to be Chris's entry into some more sexual healing, so who better than Sally to leak this information.

I blushed like a schoolgirl as I remembered my time with the new boyfriend. It had been incredible. I wasn't sure I could talk about this to Dr. Jurgens. I had read the corny Harlequin romance novels that talked about lovemaking sessions that lasted for hours. The ones that started with him nibbling your ears lobes and involved long sensuous kisses and caresses that made your skin come alive. The ones that ended in waves of pleasure with you wrapped in his arms, drifting off to sleep with your head on his chest. That is what it was like with this man.

I had truly never experienced anything like it before. He had stayed the entire night; something, as a rule I didn't let happen. A long-term relationship with another man was definitely not part of the plan. The next morning I had made us breakfast and had invited him to spend the rest of the weekend with me. It had been a weekend filled with nothing but laughter and amazing sex. I hadn't seen him since. He had an apartment in town but was working out of town and it wasn't unusual for him not be around for a couple weeks at a time. We really hadn't made any plans to get together anyway, but I was having a very hard time putting what had happened out of my head. I couldn't believe what I was feeling and realized what I had been missing all those years.

"What the hell is happening to me? I don't get it? Where is John? I'm scared, no, I'm mad! I don't want to do this. Now it's me out there, it's just wrong, what the hell is this? Now I'm going to get a sex life, after all these years—at my age? I remember begging Rick to touch me like that. Why couldn't he have made me feel that way? That's all I ever wanted from him! I just wanted him to take the time to touch me and kiss me!" I was crying. "Now along comes this guy I have never met before and in one weekend I have all of these things! I can't do this! I don't want to do this! Let Sally do this. This is Sally's thing, not mine.

"Is this what integration is all about? Where is everybody? Where is Christine? What am I supposed to do?"

"Okay, hang on, let's take a look at this," Dr. Jurgens interrupted, adding, "Do I need to really say out loud to you where you were, how bad it was, what you were ready to do? You are blowing this way out of proportion. Stop and think, clear your mind, stop and think. You can do this.

"Let's talk about the boyfriend. Sounds to me like you met a man who knows how to treat a lady in the bedroom. Also sounds like you were able to relax and enjoy the experience. You know the fact that you were able to do that in itself is not a bad thing. Do you think maybe it's okay that you're a sexual person?"

"She's doing the Miss Drama Queen thing again," Christine

said taking over, as she slid over to the edge of the couch and sat up straight. "She can get certainly get her tail in a knot."

"Hi, Christine. She seems pretty upset. This move has been hard on her. What is your take on the boyfriend?" Dr. Jurgens asked.

"Like I said, she's doing the drama queen thing, but as long as she doesn't do anything stupid . . . she still likes to blame Sally for everything, but she's doing way too much drinking and pill-popping. We would be way ahead in all this if she could get a handle on that. I can't help her when she's drinking; that shuts me down, it shuts us all down when she's drinking."

Dr. Jurgens replied, "You are right, she does need to get a handle on the drinking. That is a worry."

"Talk to her, tell her, maybe she will listen to you." Christine seemed very tired, unlike her normal confident self.

"I will," Dr. Jurgens answered, "Thanks, Christine."

Shiver and tilt. "Who was here?" I asked as I pushed my way back on the bed, grabbing the pillow and clutching it to my chest.

Dr. Jurgens answered, "Christine was here and was worried about the drinking. We need to address that," he said. "She is very worried, you know, I am not going to let up on this either. You can do this, let's get you some help for the drinking, okay?"

I knew the drinking was a problem but I enjoyed this time—the partying, the dancing, the warm, peaceful feeling. I guess I felt we deserved it after being under Rick's thumb for so long. I had myself convinced that we could keep it all under control. What was all the fuss about?

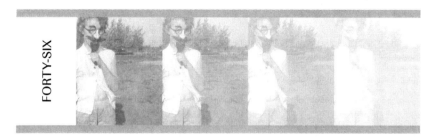

FORTY-SIX

# *Detox and the Double-V Gal*

I did address the drinking problem just like I addressed every other problem I had ever had in my life, with unrelenting determination, because that's what I did. I knew no other way; my Board of Directors knew no other way. So I did ask for help.

A week later I was admitted into a detox center. It was becoming quieter in my head. John wasn't involved in criminal activity and that was a huge relief. "Does that mean I am becoming integrated?" I had asked Dr. Jurgens when he had come to see me on the ward.

I was scared; it had been several years since I had gone a full day without my pills and, in fact, I was now "double doctoring" to get the amount I needed, something I hadn't even admitted to Dr. Jurgens. My alcohol intake had reached an all-time high. I didn't drink every day, but I was a binge drinker. I was certain to be drunk every weekend day. I told myself I would stop at two drinks but that never happened. Once I had started I could not stop. That had caused a new conflict with the alters.

John hated the alcohol and had always looked at it as a sign of weakness, as had Christine, although she had not come down so hard on Chris for it and had simply chosen to try to cover up and manage the damage, as had Elizabeth. Sally, of course, didn't have a problem with the booze but enjoyed it as part of her party scene. It was a strange scenario and one that would present itself in confusing ways and cause me a lot of conflict and misunderstanding when I did get further into the recovery program.

Admission into the detoxification center wasn't a lot different than going into the psych ward of a hospital. I thought about Jake, the huge native fellow whom I had befriended at the Villas. When I first saw him he was tied down to a bed right in view of the dining area where he most certainly went through horrible withdrawal symptoms. I wondered if I would actually have full-blown DTs and the thought of that terrified me. Watching Jake go through that, writhing and thrashing on the gurney, was horrible. The admitting nurse went through the possible things that could happen to me but she didn't think that the volume of alcohol I was ingesting would condemn me to the same fate. What they were more concerned about was the amount of lorazepam (a drug virtually the same as Valium) that I was taking. I had never realized that lorazepam and Valium were the same until this point. My addiction earned me the detox nickname the "double-V gal" because my drugs of choice were vodka and Valium.

They decided to take me off the pills gradually because of the risk of having a seizure or a stroke. That would mean going through serious drug withdrawal symptoms three times in the first ten days of treatment. This was because they gradually decreased the dosage; every time they reduced it I would go back into the withdrawal with one day in between where I would feel somewhat normal. They predicted we could do the total detox in ten days. The nurse talked to me about chills and sweats, about nausea and aching, about feeling agitated and depressed. She talked about drinking lots of water and showering frequently because the toxins evacuating from my system would cause a foul odor.

A counselor then came and got me and showed me around: the activity and chore board, the dining hall, the television room, the garden/smoke area, the meeting room, the quiet room.

Mental illness and addiction seemed to knock down all the barriers and stereotypes. There was a varied assortment of people around, no different than what you would see if you went people watching on a Saturday afternoon at the mall: two teenagers, a girl and guy; a couple of very rough-looking native men; a very good-looking middle-aged woman; a not-so good-looking middle-aged man; a couple of white men in their early thirties, one looking very pale and very sick, the other with a dirty white muscle shirt and both arms covered with tattoos; a distinguished fellow probably in his seventies also looking quite pale, but very well put together; and a couple of others I couldn't get a real good look at. I thought I heard that maximum capacity was fifteen.

The main reason for detox is getting the poison out of your system and, while that's happening, keeping your brain as busy as possible so maybe you won't notice what's happening to your body, at least that's what I had it figured out to be. Every waking minute is filled with addictions-based education: either films or presentations or meetings.

The first couple of days were not so bad. I was a little shaky. Then in the middle of the night on day three, it hit like a typhoon. I woke up and was soaked. At first I thought I wet the bed. I was freezing cold and soaking wet and the part about odor was no joke—the smell almost made me throw up. I took my bedding down to the laundry room and was getting fresh linens from the linen supply closet when the nurse on duty came up to me. There are cameras everywhere, of course, and she had seen me come in. One of their jobs was to look after linen changes but it was nearly 3:00 AM so I assumed I needed to do this myself. I must have looked wretched and I was shaking almost uncontrollably.

The nurse kindly offered to help me with my linens and in fact offered to help me take a quick shower before I went back to bed. I was so grateful I felt like crying. I was so cold and felt so dirty. It was the most awful feeling and smell. I made my way to the shower but I didn't think I could stand up. The shaking had intensified. The nurse brought me a chair, got the water running and left. The hot shower felt so good. I finally warmed up and the nurse came back and turned the water off. She wrapped a large, heated flannel sheet around me. I couldn't remember anyone ever doing anything that kind for me before. The shaking was settling down a lot and I was in new, dry pajamas. The nurse had remade my bed with fresh sheets. She wished me a good night and hoped I could get some rest. She turned the light out as she left. I hugged a pillow and rolled over, the shaking was down to a tremble now and I did feel warm. I didn't stink, but didn't smell like myself either. I must have drifted off to sleep for a while but it wasn't very long.

Then I was awake again. This time I knew I hadn't wet the bed. This time I knew what it was. The stink was back, the cold was back, and the shaking was back. I laid in the wet cold sheets, sweating, hot then cold, shaking and crying. What had I done to my body? How long would I have to do this? My arms ached. My legs ached and even my toes ached. I was going to be sick. I barely made it to the bathroom before I started to vomit. Never before had I smelled anything so vile, so putrid, so utterly rotten. I heaved and heaved until I lay on the bathroom floor, cold, shaking, empty.

Finally I pulled myself up off the tile and got back in bed. It was still wet and cold. I was cold and shaking and sick, so sick. *I should have a shower and change the sheets,* I thought. *But I can't. I feel too weak. I don't care.* I hugged my pillow and wanted to die.

No sooner had I gotten the vileness out of my stomach than I felt horrible abdominal cramping. I hurried back to the bathroom before I crapped on myself. Ten minutes later, maybe twenty, maybe a half hour—who knew—I was still sitting in the bathroom. I thought I was finished but too exhausted to even wipe, get off the toilet and make the trip to the bed.

Finally I was back in bed again. It was still damp and cold but I didn't care. I stunk and didn't care. I was sick and I hurt and I was angry and I wanted to get some sleep and I wanted a fucking drink right now! I was vibrating. The whole bed was vibrating. I hugged the pillow tighter. I had it twisted and nearly pulled it in two. I remembered some bullshit about acute withdrawal. I was ready to scream. *Breathe, remember to breath.* I was so cold.

The nurse came in to check on me and told me to come down for breakfast. This was not like a hotel; patients had to make breakfast themselves and had full use of the kitchen. "You can make anything you want," the counselor had told me, "bacon and eggs or cold cereal and a muffin—it's all up to you." I walked in and saw a selection of muffins and fresh fruit. "I can't even think about eating," I told the nurse.

She saw how sick I was. "We have to get you cleaned up," she said. "You don't have to eat anything this morning, but you have to keep drinking or you will get dehydrated." They were always talking about drinking water to flush the Valium out. I didn't care; I just wanted to clean up.

I was back in the shower and the hot water started to feel good again. My arms started to relax a little. My leg muscles quit cramping and my toes even hurt less. My stink started to flush down the drain. I was warm again and when I stepped out of the shower the nurse handed me another heated flannelette sheet and told me to rest if I could and then when I felt better, to get dressed and go down to the kitchen.

I couldn't settle in to sleep so I went down to the kitchen again. Someone was cooking bacon. It actually smelled good; not good enough to eat but decent enough that I was thinking about food again. I checked the duty board on my way by and I saw that I was on kitchen clean-up that morning. I decided on some cranberry juice, a piece of dry toast and my bottle of water. I finally took their advice about the water.

"Wowee, you look baaad!" the big native said to me with a smile. There was little point in trying to hide anything in a place like this. He added, "It must be day three or four for you."

It was all I could do to mutter back, "Three days, I think you're right." It amazed me that many of the patients had been here more than once, in fact some of them many times, and could go through this over and over again.

By the end of that day I was beginning to feel not too bad physically and that evening I actually had a regular dinner. I slept through the night without incident. I was optimistic that the worst of the detox was behind me. Then the next day they decreased my Valium.

That night, by 3:00 AM, I was on the roller coaster once more. The cold sweats, the shakes, the stink, the nausea, the diarrhea had all started again. Twenty-four hours later, when I was able to get myself together, I arrived at the nurses' station with a new plan. The original scheme had been to gradually take me off the Valium. To me that seemed to suggest I was going to have to go through one of these "stink" episodes every time they decreased it. They agreed that was the case, but was still safer once again because of the seizure and stroke risk.

I suggested another way to do this. I asked if they could take me off the Valium completely and monitor my blood pressure, and thought that maybe that would help safeguard me from the seizure and stroke risk. They agreed it would only help with the stroke issue, not the seizure, but it was still my choice. I would need to sign a waiver releasing them of their responsibility because it was going against their recommended treatment plan. They had halfway assured me the symptoms I had already experienced would be the same only likely somewhat worse taking me off the Valium completely, so the choice was go through it once worse, or go through what I had just come through twice, three, or more times.

I decided I liked the sound of "once" a whole lot better so that's what I went for. I hunkered down, expected the worst, and hoped for the best. Small mercies, the symptoms were not any worse, they just lasted an extra day. Now I could really say I was sober and straight.

Alcohol would prove to be another issue and caused a much-heated debate among the Directors. When I actually spoke at an Alcoholics Anonymous meeting in detox—they had them every day, sometimes more than once a day—and I said, "Hello, my name's Chris and I'm an alcoholic," John nearly burst a blood vessel.

"Here we fucking go! Another bandwagon! You're not an alcoholic. You just need to use a little fucking will power! First it was the fucking church, now it's going to be a fucking bunch of AA bleeding deacons. Can't you make a decision yourself? Are you always going to have someone around telling you what to do? Watch your back, because these 'too good to be true' guys, are *too good to be true! We don't need this shit; we can do this on our own!"

There was a fracas and I heard part of what was said, but I had also heard something about admitting I was powerless over alcohol. I knew I felt powerless. I wanted help. I wanted to quit drinking. I wanted to do what it took. John was of the mind that we did not need help for this, that we could do this on our own. I was glad John had taught me not to accept disrespect and abuse, I was grateful to him for that, and I was so very glad he wasn't doing anything criminal anymore; but he was wrong about this, I was pretty sure about that. I was certain I was an alcoholic. My family was full of it and you didn't end up in detox for casual drinking. I knew I could not do this without a treatment program.

So began the Board's excursion into a Twelve Step recovery program. I got off the bus from treatment and the next night attended my first meeting in town, out of the facility. I felt very welcome and looked around the room to find the friendliest, warmest, strongest faces. When it was my turn, I introduced myself as an alcoholic and told of my recent return from detox.

Sally was in the background and didn't fail to notice a couple of attractive men. John viewed everyone there with mistrust, waiting to see what their hidden agenda was. Christine, as always, was at her post; her strength would be needed here. She saw Chris as such a people-pleaser, always playing little games that someone else had made up. She hoped Chris could see she had her own strengths soon. Elizabeth liked these people; she saw them mostly as kind souls who had their own wounded hearts. She thought, *Chris would do well to find friends here—carefully mind you.* I, Chris, needed to befriend people who had learned how to heal their own wounded hearts and who could offer her amity without judgment. Elizabeth also saw this as a place for me to reestablish my faith.

Staying sober was harder than I thought it would be. I received my one-month sobriety chip and was very proud. I should have received a three-month sobriety chip. I hadn't drunk, but Sally had gone to a party after one of her good-time boyfriends called and she had fielded the phone call. She just couldn't say no.

A few weeks later I started drinking, more out of utter confusion than anything, and it wasn't long after I really should have been able to receive my three-month chip. The therapy was still continuing with Dr. Jurgens and all the alters were continuing to show up, each having their say. Alcohol was one of the major topics of conversation these days and Dr. Jurgens never let up on his concern for Chris and his absolute belief that I could not drink at all, ever again. He had also insisted I set up regular visits with an addictions counselor, which I did.

I saw the counselor every two weeks. Sally found him very handsome and likable. I also went to Dr. Jurgens once a week and three AA meetings a week, on Tuesday, Thursday and Saturday. I usually managed to get to Tuesday's meetings sober, but Thursday and Saturday would find me in various states of intoxication. Sally, the giggling flirt, attended many of those meetings, providing a lot of entertainment. I was still carrying on an intermittent relationship with the "new" boyfriend who didn't drink much but who had introduced me to marijuana and the pot-smoking crowd, hence me being high and/or intoxicated. My addictions worker had me on a waiting list to attend a twenty-eight day treatment program. Dr. Jurgens had been trying but I was very stubborn and in denial about the depth of my addiction. And so I waited.

The twenty-eight day program came and went. At least there had been no withdrawal this time. I hadn't been drinking for that long this time and had not gone back to the Valium or any other prescription medications. My days were filled with therapy; sessions on everything from STDs to post-acute withdrawal, to proper nutrition; countless, seemingly endless group meetings, listening to people tell their recovery stories; doing timelines, setting goals, on and on and on it went. Every ounce of addiction education had been pounded into my brain.

The trip home from the program was beautiful, peaceful and quiet. I was happy to have the Board of Directors with me. They had all been there with me for the program and of course all had their take on things. It was funny how they seemed to be getting along these days; they accepted and valued each other's opinions. I was looking forward to seeing Dr. Jurgens when I got back. I was anticipated going to a meeting when I returned; so did Sally and that was okay, too. John wasn't in my face about the alcoholism thing like he had been before and that was cool.

I also made a big decision: I wanted to be called Christine. It was an evolutionary sort of thing that happened when I decided to revert back to my maiden name. During therapy Dr. Jurgens asked me what I would like to be called. I said, "Christine" since I had been "Chris" my whole married life and that period was definitely over. The Board was in agreement on this. I would change my legal surname back to my maiden name. In line with that everything else changed from Chris to Christine.

This was the beginning of new strength and a major step in the integration process. It was always about acceptance and learning to value each part. Taking on Christine as my name was huge. It didn't mean devaluing Chris at all, and in fact Christine was my given name anyway, but it equated to my strength and the ability to choose my destiny. Christine was strong, smart and capable. She also had the best qualities of Chris: warmth, tenderness and compassion.

We all stayed faithful to the therapy with Dr. Jurgens, and in the subsequent years, worked at redefining who we were and what kind of life we wanted to live. Each of us by now understood the necessity of working together, of integrating. It no longer posed a threat to anyone, but it still scared us all, even John.

I suddenly realized I had all these choices, but had such little experience in making them. Luckily, I had Elizabeth, steadfast

Elizabeth. She had a good sense of character, which we all had come to appreciate. She helped me find new, loyal friends whom I could count on.

Elizabeth also gave me the direction and the courage to connect with a new church family and the understanding that God had never left my side. A spiritual healing slowly and wonderfully unfolded.

The healing process continued and layer by layer, bit by bit, each member of the Board came to feel comfortable with the part they had played in this life, so comfortable that I hadn't heard from any of them, individually, in awhile. I wasn't even sure how long that was. It was a subtle, quiet merging. There was no "integration day" and *poof*, everyone was gone. I was simply aware that there was a strange but peaceful quiet in my head.

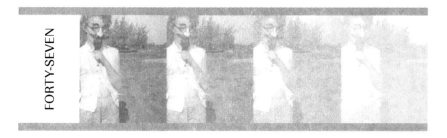

FORTY-SEVEN

# *Full Circle*

More and more, as the weeks of therapy had unraveled, I had felt a certain yearning to revisit where it had all started. This desire grew until I could no longer ignore it: I had to go back. I wasn't sure why, I just felt compelled to make this journey. I called Karen and Kevin, two of my closest friends in my new life, because I knew this was not a trip I could—or should—take alone. It was a thirty-four mile drive from Merrimore to my home farm site. We filled in the long stretch of highway with small talk, which helped quell some of my anxiety. It was a very dull grey day and occasionally it seemed like it was going to rain. I was glad. It felt right that the sun wasn't shining for this day.

When we got to Riverdale I pointed out the church I had attended. It was right on the highway on the edge of town. We continued past it. I had little to no feelings about that church. What a strange thing. I had worked so hard there and devoted so much time, only to be ostracized. But rehashing that episode really wasn't what this trip was about. We drove further on the same highway, not even a mile along was the home I had built after the fire, and I pointed it out to my friends. It was a beautiful house and was only three years old when I left it behind. I still felt little to nothing. That was not what this trip was about either.

We turned onto a gravel road and started out into the country and then things started to change. This was the same gravel road I traveled as a girl on a yellow school bus for twelve years. I started to go back in time. I directed Karen to stop at a corner and I explained that this was my bus stop. Just down from this corner was where my dad's cousin lived—the one I was sure my dad had molested in the granary. My family home farmyard was visible from here and as we drove further the white story-and-a-half house came into view. My heart pounded faster. It was so loud I could hear it. We turned into the driveway. The place was much different than I remembered. The entire row of natural growth trees was gone. The new owners had planted other trees that were just saplings. The yard looked bare, desolate. There were no fences or farm outbuildings. The barn and granary were gone. There was just a house and a garage. We sat in the truck for a minute.

"Maybe we should just go, this is enough," I said and I tried to describe things from inside the truck. It was a lame attempt. I knew I *needed* to get out of the truck but now that I was here I was filled with anxiety. "I don't want to get out of the truck. I heard the owner was cranky and would think we were trespassing," I said, hoping they would agree.

"No, we need to get out," Kevin said.

I took a deep breath, knowing he would not let me back out. "I will ask if it's okay to look around," I said.

I went to the house, introduced myself, and asked if it was okay to look around outside. "Why sure, take your time," she said graciously. Karen and Kevin get out of the truck and for a minute or two I just walked around the yard alone.

The yard had changed immensely, even since Rick and I had lived here. The new owners had cleared out all the natural forest, cultivated it and planted new trees in perfect rows. That made the house stand out, looking big and lonely. The forest had provided such a beautiful backdrop before. Now everything seemed exposed.

I tried to think about where things were. As I walked toward where the row of trees used to be I came to a dead stop. I found myself standing at the edge of a hollow in the earth where the out-house had been. I had walked right to it, just like I had a hundred times when I was a little girl. There had been no hesitation. Kevin and Karen had followed me. I pointed to it. I just stood there. For an instant we all stood there. There was no doubt about it. This was it. Kevin said something but I couldn't comprehend it. He walked away. I felt his anger. But there was no more anger for me. That was gone. Karen stood beside me, trembling.

It was so green and alive; there were pretty little white flow-ers right in the middle of the hollow in the ground and an aspen seedling had sprouted. There was fresh grass, glistening from the light rain that has just started and tiny new poplar trees growing. I felt the wind come up. I closed my eyes and leaned back and let it blow over my face. It was cool, crisp and clean. There was no evil here anymore. I wanted my friends to know that. It could not hurt me anymore.

"There is no power here," I said to my friends who stood on either side of me. I became aware of how quiet it was in my head and a sob started somewhere deep in my soul. It was okay; its time had come. I placed an arm around Kevin and Karen and I let that cry rise to the surface. I felt the cool spring rain that had just started mix with my tears and I held on tight to my friends.

We got back in the car and drove further down the road to where Grandpa and Grandma lived, the yard where I had the wonder-ful picnics with Great-Grandma Annie and the mysterious Uncle John. At the end of that road we turned around in the yard where Larry's family had once lived. All that was left of his house was a skeleton. We drove back past my home yard and I asked Karen to stop for a minute.

"One more look," I said. "I don't think I am ever going to be back." My eyes took it all in and then we drove off.

It was very quiet in the truck. After a while I announced that I was proud of myself because I didn't split to do this and I didn't buy any booze. It was quiet again, the tears welled up in my eyes and I let them fall. Karen drove slowly and cried softly. Kevin sat in the back seat. He slid forward and placed his hand on my shoulder. We stayed that way for many miles, each with our own thoughts. As we drove I wondered, *Do they know? Do they understand that something beautiful has happened today? Is there some way I can tell them?* There was such peace. The evil was truly gone.

In the same row of trees where so much horror was dealt out, the Northern Lights touched down again and again until I was fully engulfed in God's goodness and I heard the voices of a thousand angels through that very same row of trees. And now on this same spot, I embraced a friendship that held the same kind of beauty. I wondered where these two souls came from, and then was simply grateful they were here with me. I hoped that they knew how much their support meant to me.

# Epilogue

Twelve years after I discovered the horrible truth of my childhood, the hurricane of this reality blew through my mind and I was left to clean up the pieces. It was arduous and often traumatizing. To get better I had to relive the past and it often set me back. Healing required time and patience but the years of difficult work in therapy paid off and I achieved what many people with my condition do not: integration. It wasn't like New Year's Day where you go to sleep in one year and wake up in another; I didn't go to bed one night with the several personalities and wake up the next morning with just one. Neither was it a "peeling off" and disappearance of people—like the children singing "so long, farewell" in *The Sound of Music.* Instead it was a gradual melting together of many into one.

This analogy from my childhood might offer insight into this process. When I was six or seven years old we had a big iron, wood-burning stove that served a dual purpose: as a way to cook and also to heat our small home. Once, I was sitting near the stove—which had cooled off enough to be safe to sit next to it—coloring with my new box of eight crayons. One happened to come in contact with the stove and I watched the line that I had drawn melt. It was a strange and wonderful transformation. My blue crayon had turned into a beautiful waterfall. I was fascinated by this and took out another color, drawing a wavy line above the blue one; it was so pretty. I took another color and another and another; with each one I drew a line above the previous one. The colors flowed into one another, creating entirely new shades.

Just as those colors had mixed to become a new color, and those original hues could never be separated again, so it was with my integration. As the personalities melted together they formed something different that could not be divided.

There is still so much controversy over the diagnosis of DID. People often ask me questions like: How does this happen in the first place? If I talk to myself, do I have it? As Dr. Jurgens explained to me, dissociation is normal and it operates on a continuum ranging from mild to extreme. It is the ability, in some way, to move ourselves aside. If you have ever pulled into your driveway at night after work and wondered how you got there, then you have dissociated. Your mind is so used to the daily drive that you went on autopilot to get home. To the right of that on the scale might be the teenager who is bored in physics class and mentally checks out during the lecture. Further on down the continuum is the woman who forgets the pain of childbirth when deciding to increase the size of her family. As the continuum moves right the triggers to dissociate are more pronounced. A child may be upset by his parents' constant conflict; he moves back from it mentally and emotionally, not really hearing the screaming anymore. dissociative identity disorder weighs in on the far right side of the continuum. The experience, the pain, is so severe, beyond anything that the brain can handle, and so it dissociates.

My alters, my Board of Directors, helped me through the trauma of abuse almost like runners in a relay race. Each did his or her part and carried the baton for my team. When they were gone, I had to run the whole length of the track each and every day by myself—and that was daunting for me. I missed them. Sometimes I would actually try to will them back but it didn't happen. That feeling subsided with time and with acceptance of my new reality.

There is quiet in my head now. Sometimes I awaken during the night and the silence is deafening. It has been over four years since my full integration and I have to admit that the first year or so I was sometimes frightened by the intense stillness. The Board had been such a big part of my life, constantly talking to and guiding me, that I went through a grieving process of sorts when they were gone. Though they often visited havoc and mayhem upon my life because they did not have a full perspective on it, they were my reality and I missed them. As the saying goes, the devil you know is better than the devil you don't know.

Life, by definition, is challenging and because the experience of living integrated was uncharted territory for me, I was initially unsure how to handle the daily issues, big and small. Eventually I came to realize that though the actual personalities were gone they left me with their strengths and abilities. I became grateful for the part each of them had played in helping a defenseless little girl survive and in making me into the woman I am now—and the one I am still becoming:

John taught me how to respect myself and not allow anyone to abuse me in anyway;

Sally showed me the wonderful side of being feminine and sexual without shame and embarrassment;

Elizabeth restored my faith and gave me an appreciation for the beauty and wonder of all God's creation;

Chris helped me realize that compassion and empathy are not weaknesses but strengths; and finally

Christine, with her intellect and composure, taught me that learning and growth are possible no matter how old you are.

I know without a doubt that I could not have accomplished any of this without help. My strong support system has made all the difference in the world. I have family, friends, and professionals who have walked every step of the way with me and will continue to do so in the future.

My integration has been tested by alcohol relapses, family dilemmas, and "life" in general. There is no going back, no calling the Board for help, and no creating new alters. Has it been easy? Hell, no! But it has been worth it. I was given the choice of hauling my past around with me like a sack of rocks or to put it down and walk away. I chose to walk away. I can't change it so I walk in forgiveness both of my perpetrators and myself. I embrace integration with a huge portion of gratitude.

I don't mind the quiet now; in fact some mornings it takes me a few extra minutes to get out of bed because I bask in the safety of the stillness.

It is my prayer that my story can offer encouragement and hope for those suffering. It is my desire that you read these words and find the voice you need to ask for help. You are worth it.

# About the Author

Christine Ducommun is enjoying her retirement—from working and especially from therapy. She takes immense pleasure in her new quiet life. She takes part in many social activities as well as the abundant festivals, programs, and special events in the city in which she lives.

Concerned about the stigma that still attaches itself to mental health issues, she plans to advocate on a volunteer basis for those affected. Mostly, her life is about peace and harmony: no more rush and fuss, no more chaos, but simply being open to where God leads.

To contact: www.ChristineDucommun.com.

# Other Books by
# Bettie Youngs Book Publishers

## The Maybelline Story
## And the Spirited Family Dynasty Behind It

### Sharrie Williams

A woman's most powerful possession is a man's imagination.
**—Maybelline ad, 1934**

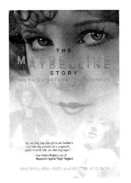

In 1915, when a kitchen-stove fire singed his sister Mabel's lashes and brows, Tom Lyle Williams watched in fascination as she performed what she called "a secret of the harem"—mixing petroleum jelly with coal dust and ash from a burnt cork and applying it to her lashes and brows. Mabel's simple beauty trick ignited Tom Lyle's imagination, and he started what would become a billion-dollar business, one that remains a viable American icon after nearly a century. He named it Maybelline in her honor.

Throughout the twentieth century, the Maybelline company inflated, collapsed, endured, and thrived in tandem with the nation's upheavals. Williams—to avoid unwanted scrutiny of his private life—cloistered himself behind the gates of his Rudolph Valentino Villa and ran his empire from a distance. Now, after nearly a century of silence, this true story celebrates the life of an American entrepreneur, a man whose vision rocketed him to success along with the woman held in his orbit: Evelyn Boecher—who became his lifelong fascination and muse. Captivated by her "roaring charisma," he affectionately called her the "real Miss Maybelline" and based many of his advertising campaigns on the woman she represented: commandingly beautiful, hard-boiled, and daring. Evelyn masterminded a life of vanity, but would fall prey to fortune hunters and a mysterious murder that even today remains unsolved.

A fascinating and inspiring story, a tale both epic and intimate, alive with the clash, the hustle, the music, and dance of American enterprise.

A richly told juicy story of a forty-year, white-hot love triangle that fans the flames of a major worldwide conglomerate.
**—Neil Shulman, associate producer,** *Doc Hollywood*

ISBN: 978-0-9843081-1-8 • $18.95

In bookstores everywhere, online, or from the publisher:
www.BettieYoungsBooks.com

# *Out of the Transylvania Night*

### *Aura Imbarus*

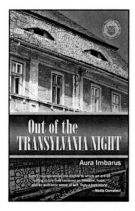

An epic tale of identity, love, and the indomitable human spirit.

Communist dictator Nicolae Ceaușescu had turned Romania into a land of zombies as surely as if Count Dracula had sucked its lifeblood. Yet Aura Imbarus dares to be herself: a rebel among the gray-clad, fearful masses. Christmas shopping in 1989, Aura draws sniper fire as Romania descends into the violence of a revolution that topples one of the most draconian regimes in the Soviet bloc. With a bit of Hungarian mysticism in her blood, astonishingly accurate visions lead Aura into danger—as well as to the love of her life. They marry and flee a homeland still in chaos. With only two pieces of luggage and a powerful dream, they settle in Los Angeles where freedom and sudden wealth challenge their love as powerfully as Communist tyranny.

Aura loses her psychic vision, heirloom jewels are stolen, a fortune is lost, followed by divorce. But their early years as lovers in a war-torn country and their rich family heritage is the glue that reunites them. They pay a high price for their materialistic dreams, but gain insight and a love that is far richer. *Out of the Transylvania Night* is a deftly woven narrative about finding greater meaning and fulfillment in both free and closed societies.

Aura's courage shows the degree to which we are all willing to live lives centered on freedom, hope, and an authentic sense of self. Truly a love story!
**—Nadia Comaneci, Olympic gold medalist**

If you grew up hearing names like Tito, Mao, and Ceaușescu but really didn't understand their significance, read this book!
**—Mark Skidmore, Paramount Pictures**

This book is sure to find its place in memorial literature of the world.
**—Beatrice Ungar, editor-in-chief, Hermannstädter Zeitung**

ISBN: 978-0-9843081-2-5 • $14.95

In bookstores everywhere, online, or from the publisher:
www.BettieYoungsBooks.com

# On Toby's Terms

## Charmaine Hammond

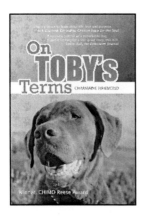

When Charmaine and her husband adopted Toby, a five-year-old Chesapeake Bay retriever, they figured he might need some adjusting time, but they certainly didn't count on what he'd do in the meantime. Soon after he entered their lives and home, Toby proved to be a holy terror who routinely opened and emptied the hall closet, turned on water taps, pulled and ate things from the bookshelves, sat for hours on end in the sink, and spent his days rampaging through the house. Oddest of all was his penchant for locking himself in the bathroom, and then pushing the lid of the toilet off the tank, smashing it to pieces. After a particularly disastrous encounter with the knife-block in the kitchen—and when the couple discovered Toby's bloody paw prints on the phone—they decided Toby needed professional help. Little did they know what they would discover about this dog.

*On Toby's Terms* is an endearing story of a beguiling creature who teaches his owners that, despite their trying to teach him how to be the dog they want, he is the one to lay out the terms of being the dog he needs to be. This insight would change their lives forever.

Simply a beautiful book about life, love, and purpose.
　　　**—Jack Canfield, Coauthor** *Chicken Soup for the Soul* **series**

In a perfect world, every dog would have a home and every home would have a dog—like Toby!
　　　**—Nina Siemaszko, actress,** *The West Wing*

This is a captivating, heartwarming story and we are very excited about bringing it to film.
　　　**—Steve Hudis, Producer, IMPACT Motion Pictures**

ISBN: 978-0-9843081-4-9 • $14.95

In bookstores everywhere, online, or from the publisher:
www.BettieYoungsBooks.com

## Blackbird Singing in the Dead of Night
## What to Do When God Won't Answer

### Gregory L. Hunt

*"Blackbird singing in the dead of night,*
*take these broken wings and learn to fly…"* —The Beatles

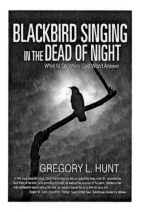

Pastor Greg Hunt had devoted nearly thirty years to congregational ministry, helping people experience God and find their way in life. Then came his own crisis of faith and calling. While turning to God for guidance, he finds nothing. Neither his education—a Ph.D. in theology—nor his religious involvements—senior pastor of a multi-staff congregation, and a civic and denominational leader—could prepare him for the disorienting impact of the experience.

Days turned into months. Months became seasons. Seasons added up to a year, then two. He began to wonder if his faith had been an illusion. Was God even real? In the midst of his struggle, he tries a desperate experiment in devotion: Could he have a personal encounter with God through the red letters of Jesus, as recorded in the Gospel of Matthew?

The result is startling—and changes his life entirely.

Sometimes raw, always honest, and ultimately hopeful, *Blackbird Singing in the Dead of Night* speaks to the spiritual longings of the human heart. **—Julie Pennington-Russell, senior pastor, First Baptist Church, Decatur, GA**

In this most beautiful memoir, Greg Hunt invites us into an unsettling time in his life, exposes the fault lines of his faith, and describes the path he walked into and out of the dark. Thanks to the trail markers he leaves along the way, he makes it easier for us to find our way, too.

**—Susan M. Heim, co-author,**
*Chicken Soup for the Soul, Devotional Stories for Women*

ISBN: 978-1-936332-07-6 • $15.95

In bookstores everywhere or from the publisher:
www.BettieYoungsBooks.com

# Amazing Adventures of a Nobody

### Leon Logothetis

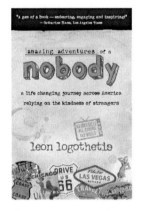

In a time of economic anxiety, global terror and shaken confidence, Englishman Leon Logothetis, star of the hit series *Amazing Adventures of a Nobody* (National Geographic Channels International, Fox Reality), shows us what is good about mankind: the simple calling people have to connect to others.

Tired of his disconnected life and uninspiring job, Leon Logothetis leaves it all behind—job, money, home, even his cell phone—and hits the road with nothing but the clothes on his back and five dollars in his pocket. His journey from Times Square to the Hollywood sign relying on the kindness of strangers and the serendipity of the open road, inspire a dramatic and life-changing transformation.

Along the way, Leon offers up the intriguing and charming tales gathered along his one-of-a-kind journey: riding in trains, buses, big rigs and classic cars; sleeping on streets and couches and firehouses; meeting pimps and preachers, astronauts and single moms, celebrities and homeless families, veterans and communists.

Each day of his journey, we catch sight of the invisible spiritual underpinning of society in these stories of companionship—and sheer adventure—that prove that the kind, good soul of mankind has not been lost.

A gem of a book: endearing, engaging and inspiring!
**—Catharine Hamm,** *Los Angeles Times*, **travel editor**

Masterful storytelling! Leon begins his journey as a merry prankster and ends a grinning philosopher. Really funny—and insightful, too.
**—Karen Salmansohn, AOL Career Coach,**
**and Oprah.com Relationship Columnist**

ISBN: 978-0-9843081-3-2 • $14.95

In bookstores everywhere, online, or from the publisher:
www.BettieYoungsBooks.com

# It Started with Dracula
## The Count, My Mother, and Me

### *Jane Congdon*

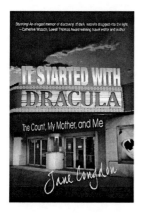

The terrifying legend of Count Dracula, silently skulking through the Transylvania night may have terrified generations of filmgoers, but the tall, elegant vampire captivated and electrified a young Jane Congdon, igniting a dream to one day see his mysterious land of ancient castles and misty hollows.

Four decades later, she finally takes her long-awaited trip—never dreaming that it would unearth decades-buried memories of life with an alcoholic mother. Set in Dracula's backyard, the story unfolds in a mere eighteen days as the author follows the footsteps of Dracula from Bucharest to the Carpathian Mountains and the Black Sea. Dracula's legend becomes the prism through which she revisits her childhood, and lays claim to a happiness she had never known.

A memoir full of surprises, Jane's story is one of hope, love—and second chances.

Unfinished business can surface when we least expect it. *It Started with Dracula* is the inspiring story of two parallel journeys: one a carefully planned vacation and the other an astonishing and unexpected detour in healing a wounded heart.

**—Charles Whitfield, MD, bestselling author of**
*Healing the Child Within*

An elegant memoir of discovery, of dark secrets dragged into the light.
**—Catherine Watson, Lowell Thomas**
**Award-winning travel editor and author**

An elegantly written and cleverly told real-life adventure story, proving that the struggle for self-love is universal. An electrifying read.
**—Diane Bruno, CISION Media**

ISBN: 978-1-936332-10-6 • $15.95

In bookstores everywhere, online, or from the publisher:
www.BettieYoungsBooks.com

# *Diary of a Beverly Hills Matchmaker*

### *Marla Martenson*

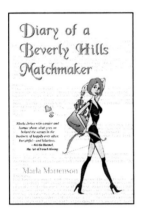

The inside scoop from the Cupid of Beverly Hills, who has brought together countless couples who have gone on to live happily ever after. But for every success story there are ridiculously funny dating disasters with high-maintenance, out-of-touch, impossible to please, dim-witted clients!

Marla takes her readers for a hilarious romp through her days as an L.A. matchmaker and her daily struggles to keep her self-esteem from imploding in a town where looks are everything and money talks. From juggling the demands her out-of-touch clients, to trying her best to meet the capricious demands of an insensitive boss, to the ups and downs of her own marriage to a Latin husband who doesn't think that she is "domestic" enough, Marla writes with charm and self-effacement about the universal struggles all women face in their lives. Readers will laugh, cringe, and cry as they journey with her through outrageous stories about the indignities of dating in Los Angeles, dealing with overblown egos, vicariously hobnobbing with celebrities, and navigating the wannabe-land of Beverly Hills. In a city where perfection is almost a prerequisite, even Marla can't help but run for the BOTOX every once in a while.

Marla's quick wit will have you rolling on the floor.
—**Megan Castran, international YouTube Queen**

Sharper than a Louboutin stiletto, Martenson's book delivers!
—**Nadine Haobsh,** *Beauty Confidential*

Martenson's irresistible wit is not to be missed.
—**Kyra David, author,** *Lust, Loathing, and a Little Lip Gloss*

ISBN: 978-0-9843081-0-1 • $14.95

In bookstores everywhere, online, or from the publisher:
www.BettieYoungsBooks.com

# Hostage of Paradox: A Memoir

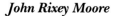

## *John Rixey Moore*

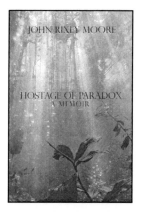

A profound odyssey of a young college graduate who enlists in the military to avoid being drafted, becomes a Green Beret Airborne Ranger, and is sent to Vietnam where he is plunged into high-risk, deep-penetration operations under contract to the CIA-work for which he was neither specifically trained nor psychologically prepared, yet for which he is ultimately highly decorated.

His life in the cloying embrace of the jungle, where even the prettiest flowers are poisonous, becomes a paradoxical labyrinth: the hard-learned language of the jungle's sounds speaks equally to both sides, the verdant canopy acts both as cover and a hazard enabling the enemy to work in close; the missions are given as important, yet the war is pointless. Moore survives his combat assignments by the thinnest measure of improbabilities. But survives he does.

Upon his return, he seeks sanctuary in a Scottish monastery and then works as a rock drill operator in a large industrial gold mine in Canada, and ultimately a career in television and film.

A compelling story told with extraordinary insight, disconcerting reality, and engaging humor.
—**David Hadley, actor,** *China Beach,* *Quantum Leap*

An epic tale!
—**Cliff Potts, actor,** *Once an Eagle,*
*Silent Running,* **and** *Wild Hearts*

Intensely personal and perceptive. You'll never forget this book! Simply the best Vietnam narrative I have ever read.
—**Leon Logothetis, host, producer, best-selling author,**
*Amazing Adventures of a Nobody*

ISBN: 978-1-936332-37-3 • $18.95

In bookstores everywhere, online, or from the publisher:
www.BettieYoungsBooks.com

# DON CARINA

### Ron Russell

*Southern Italy in the 1930s was chaotic and violent-the rise of dictator Mussolini, the dawn of Europe's descent into another World War, and continuation of turf battles between Mafia families. This was certainly no place for a young woman to assume power, but seventeen-year-old Carina would have no choice in the matter.*

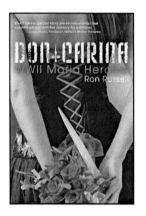

A father's death in Southern Italy in the 1930s-a place where women who can read are considered unfit for marriage-thrusts seventeen-year-old Carina into servitude as a "black widow," a legal head of the household who cares for her twelve younger siblings. A scandal forces her into a marriage to Russo, the "Prince of Naples." As head of the mafia, or Camorra, he turns her seven younger brothers into criminals.

Her black widow skills prove invaluable to Russo, and his enterprise prospers, until Mussolini allies with the Nazi Germany war machine. With three children under the age of seven, the Russo family faces food shortages, martial law under the Gestapo, and devastating Allied air raids.

One night, a bomb rips through their house causing Russo to lose his mind and start babbling secrets. If the Camorra learns of this, Carina knows an ensuing turf war will rob her of her home, her life, and the lives of everyone dear to her.

By cunning force, Carina seizes control of Russo's organization and uses her skill and savvy to control the most powerful of Mafia groups. Discovery is inevitable-and, Interpol has been watching as well. Nevertheless, Carina survives to tell her children her stunning story of strength and survival.

978-0-9843081-9-4 • $15.95

In bookstores everywhere, online, or from the publisher:
www.BettieYoungsBooks.com

# Bettie Youngs Books

*We specialize in MEMOIRS
. . . books that celebrate
fascinating people and
remarkable journeys*

VISIT OUR WEBSITE AT
www.BettieYoungsBooks.com

CPSIA information can be obtained at www.ICGtesting.com
Printed in the USA
LVOW062049040912

297341LV00001B/8/P